AFTER YOUR CHILD'S DIAGNOSIS

A PRACTICAL GUIDE FOR FAMILIES RAISING CHILDREN WITH DISABILITIES

by

Cathy Lynn Binstock, LMSW-ACP

E.M. Press, Inc.
Manassas, VA

Copyright © 1997 by Cathy Lynn Binstock
First Edition
Cover design: Adoracíon, by Colombian-born painter Orlando Agudelo-Botero. Multi-media painting on canvas, 72" x 48", 1990. Represented by Engman International, Coral Gables, FL 33134
All rights reserved. No part of this book may be reproduced or utilized in any form or by any means, electronic or mechanical, including photocopying, or by any information storage and retrieval system without permission in writing from the publisher.

ISBN: 1-880664-21-6
Library of Congress Catalog Card Number: 97-16991

E.M. Press, Inc.
P.O. Box 4057
Manassas, VA 20108

Contents

Prologue 1
Chapter One 8
   The Road Toward Acceptance
Chapter Two 19
   The Grieving Process
Chapter Three 35
   The Marriage
Chapter Four 43
   The Siblings
Chapter Five 50
   The Grandparents/Extended Family
Chapter Six 56
   Fostering Independence for Children with Disabilities
Chapter Seven 68
   Issues for Adolescents with Disabilities
Chapter Eight 78
   The School
Chapter Nine 91
   Future Planning
Chapter Ten 96
   Adults with Disabilities Living Meaningful Lives
Chapter Eleven 113
   Single Parents

Chapter Twelve 120
    Alternative Care

Glossary 123
Resource Guide 129
Bibliography 155

Acknowledgements

A special heartfelt thanks to all the families, children and adults who participated in this project.

My gratitude to all the professionals and agencies throughout the United States who helped distribute questionnaires and provide guidance:

Johnnie Maloy of the Houston Council of San Jacinto Girl Scouts, Houston, Texas
Marguerite Priest of the Challenger Division Little League, Houston, Texas
Ricky Rainville of the YMCA at Lake Houston, Kingwood, Texas
Dr. Nancy Robinson, Webster, Texas
Gail Goodwin of Our Kids Magazine, Houston, Texas
Tom Dibello of Dynamic Orthotics, Houston, Texas
Hope Center for Therapy at Moody Gardens, Galveston, Texas
Monique Miller of Bay Area Rehabilitation Center, Houston, Texas
Take Notice of the Houston Chronicle, Houston, Texas
Louise Horst of Therapeutic Alliance, Houston, Texas
Developmental Steps, Houston, Texas
Nancy Ward of the Transition Learning Center, Webster, Texas
Terri Phillips-Whitman, M.S., L.M.S.W.-A.C.P., Houston, Texas
Dr. Peter M. Levine, Houston, Texas
Dr. Ken Kopel, Houston, Texas
Dr. Jean Lerner, Houston, Texas
Linda Horton of the Early Childhood Intervention Center, Denison, Texas

Elaine Hime, Houston, Texas
Eve Cugini of Family to Family Support Group, Houston, Texas
Tony Koosis of the Houston Independent Living Center, Houston, Texas
Suzanne Cuthbertson of Arbor School, Houston, Texas
Mark Brown of Disability Rights Education Defense Fund, Berkeley, California
Richard Gorman of Estate Planning Program for Disabilities, Boulder, Colorado
Larry Foreman of Comprehensive Rehabilitation Consultants, Miami, Florida
Ginny Thornburgh of the National Organization on Disability, Washington, D.C.
Patrick Hayes for North American Riders of the Handicapped Association, Denver, Colorado
Leslie Jackson of the Pediatric Program, Bethesda, Maryland
American Occupational Therapy Association, Rockville, Maryland
Regi Boem of Team Talk, Milwaukee, Wisconsin
Fritzi Doriean of Bay-Arenac Intermediate School District of Bay City, Michigan
Jan Johnson of Colerain School, Columbus, Ohio
Sharon Gage of Parent Resource Specialists, Belleville, Illinois
Coordinating Council for Handicapped Children, Chicago, Illinois
Bruce Eddy of American Association of University, Affiliated Programs for Persons with Developmental Disabilities, Silver Springs, Maryland
Long Island Parenting News, New York, New York
United Cerebral Palsy, New York, New York
The National Parent Network, Alexandria, Virginia

To my daughters, Brooke, Melissa and Samantha.
To my husband, Bob.
To my faithful family—My mother who spent countless hours typing and revising the manuscript, my stepfather, sisters and grandmother.
To my friends who stood by our family.
To my editors, Ellen Beck and Cindy Cross, for believing in this project.

Acknowledgements

To my publisher, Beth Miller, for her support.

To my friend, Orlando Agudelo-Botero, for providing his artistic expression and dedication.

To Dr. James Gage, Dr. Carlos Rivera and Jane Leonard for giving me hope.

Prologue

Samantha's milestones were delayed. She was unable to sit up the way most babies did; she crawled very late and she was not able to walk. I was told repeatedly by our pediatrician that "she'd get there," when I asked why she seemed to be behind the other children. I guess I suspected there was a problem very early on but hoped I was wrong.

By the time she turned fifteen months old, she was unable to stand or walk. I knew something was wrong. I consulted an orthopedic surgeon, and he diagnosed her with a neurological problem and referred me to a pediatric neurologist. I left his office in tears.

The next week changed my life forever. Samantha was diagnosed with static encephalopathy. She was fitted for a leg brace, prescribed physical therapy twice a week and referred to Mental Health, Mental Retardation Association, for an infant stimulation class.

The explanations to family and friends became so painful I eventually stopped taking calls. The beginning was a time to piece together information. I went to the library, the bookstore and the medical library looking for any information I could find about static encephalopathy. I couldn't find those words anywhere. I finally discovered them in a pediatric neurology book. Under static encephalopathy, this is what I found: "Cerebral palsy - a disorder of movement and posture due to defect or lesion of the immature brain. The term cerebral palsy is not favored among pediatric neurologists, partly due to its lack of specificity, partly due to its pejorative connotation. Since the term is firmly ingrained in the medical literature and is utilized widely in the general community, there is little point in attempting to remove it. However, for purposes of clarity, pediatric neurologists currently utilize the term static encephalopathy. As a group, individuals with static encephalopathy are among the most severely handicapped and because of their motor disability, are readily identifiable by others."[1]

And so, I sat in the middle of the bookstore floor, sobbing. That moment of understanding was the most terrifying moment of my life. I could only imagine a 'crippled child', a stereotypical picture of a person with a disability. My child was disabled.

A developmental disability is a severe, chronic, mental or physical impairment that occurs before the person reaches age twenty-two—the developmental years. This substantially limits the person's abilities in such things as self-care, language, learning, physical mobility, self-direction, ability to live independently and economic self-sufficiency. Cerebral palsy is one of the most common physical disabilities of childhood. It is a non-progressive disorder characterized by abnormal coordination and muscle tone, resulting in increased spasticity and impairment of motor function. Approximately 700,000 Americans manifest some degree of CP and one-third are under the age of twenty-one. CP is a catch-all term used to describe virtually any difficulty with coordinated movement and posture caused by a brain injury.

I went through the next few months in a numb, mechanical state. I remember the first few weeks at Texas Children's Hospital where Samantha had physical therapy. I remember watching other parents who seemed to be at ease or at least coping better than I was. I had never seen so many children in wheelchairs, with walkers and canes, wearing braces. I had entered a world I never knew existed. I vividly remember one mother and her brown-haired daughter. The child must have been around five years old. She was brightly dressed, sitting in a very small wheelchair, which had been trimmed with colorful stickers and neon pink stripes. On her legs were clear-colored plastic braces. Her mother was trying to brush her hair while the child's head shook involuntarily in a seizure-like way, from side to side. All the while, the woman was having a normal chitchat with the receptionist while putting a red barrette in the little girl's hair. I quickly turned in embarrassment when

Prologue

they saw me watching. Silently screaming, I wanted to say, "How do you get used to this? How am I ever going to learn to live with this?"

My daily carefree routine was quickly replaced with medical appointments and reading anything I could find to try to help my family adjust. Everything changed. I even lost my name. Some professionals began calling me "Mom." Some referred to my daughter as a "little hemi," short for hemiplegia. What happened to our identity as people? Some professionals, however, offered support and kindness. I remember fitting Samantha for braces five times with no luck and wanting to give up. Our orthotist, Tom, said, "I'll find one to fit her, don't be discouraged." This kindness helped.

I searched for answers everywhere. I visited my rabbi, a psychiatrist and a psychologist. I read spiritual anthologies; I scanned every church bulletin board, the ones with the philosophical daily message...and I'm Jewish! I went through the classic "why me?" stuff. I received well-intentioned advice, both solicited and unsolicited. Everything helped but nothing helped. I was in deep grief and I knew it was slow-going from here.

I felt that no one understood the depth of my pain. People meant well and tried to provide comfort. They were hurting for me as well. In the beginning, many people told me to take care of myself and my own needs. I knew they were trying to tell me to look after myself so I could manage the challenging demands. But I took offense at this remark. I was barely hanging on, let alone meeting my needs. Some even said, "You have to get on with your life." In the midst of grief, that wasn't exactly the most comforting thing to hear. The worst comment had to be, "You should feel fortunate, her case is only mild." Well, to me, having mild cerebral palsy wasn't like having mild chicken pox. I certainly didn't see how fortunate I was. Again, well-intentioned people would say, "You're handling this so well." Meanwhile, I was crying everyday and was anxiety-ridden. Some said, thinking it was a compliment, "God knew what he was doing when he gave Samantha to you." Okay, I wasn't the "Mom" anymore, I was a saint—spare me this role, please. One time, I told someone that our family was learning sign language to help Samantha communicate, and the person responded with, "How neat!" I didn't know that sign language was like buying a new dress. After a while, I started pulling away. I walked in two worlds.

In the midst of the chaos, I was wanting some normal routine so I took my van to the car wash. I ran into the rabbi from my older daughters' school. He asked about the baby and if I had met any families with similar problems for support. I told him that I wasn't ready for that yet. I explained that others told me that our family should feel fortunate because Samantha's case was considered mild. I began to cry. He put his hand on my shoulder and said, "I know you don't feel very fortunate right now." That moment of another's acknowledging of my despair is something I haven't forgotten.

My other children said some funny things about Samantha. But they also became sensitive to her needs. At the grocery store, and out of the blue, my six-year-old daughter, Melissa, told Peggy, the cashier, that "Samantha had a weird brain." She couldn't just say it softly. She yelled it and repeated it so that it became a chant. Everyone around us heard her. I wanted to put the paper sack over my head and leave. As time went on, the girls started to learn more about Samantha's disabilities. My six-year-old asked the librarian at school to help her find books about disabilities. She also chose her little sister for her "treasure," which was an art project topic. My eight-year-old daughter read an article about therapeutic horseback riding to her class.

The essence of my being unraveled, my sorrow, so intense at times, seemed impossible to reconcile with the routine of daily life. My hope was to somehow defy the neurologist's diagnosis. My deep denial only led to the unjust reality.

Families living with disabilities must quickly develop survival skills to learn to live with the unknown. Existing in a sea of unanswered questions is compounded with a constant state of anxiety. Everything that once seemed stable crumbles away.

Our family, like so many others, faced a whirlwind of emotion. We felt guilty, that we were to blame. We felt anxious about needing to plan for the future and wanting more knowledge than we were given. We resented the great demands on our time. Our other children felt left out and demanded our attention. Slowly, as everything around me was changing, so did I. I dropped prior

Prologue

volunteer commitments, closed my office, dropped out of play group, shopped in places where I wouldn't have to answer questions from people who knew me. I isolated myself. I had to. I camped out at my mother and stepdad's house on the weekends. They were the only ones who really understood my pain. I threw away my big leather appointment book, and replaced it with a flowery Hallmark-looking calendar with only a small space under the date for "daily to-do things." I unconsciously began living one day at a time.

My romantic once-a-week dinners out with my husband turned into heartbreaking assessments of Samantha's extremely slow progress. And on every one of these dates one of us would cry. In the beginning, my husband was very slow to respond and accept the severity of the situation. This only increased my sense of isolation. When he did finally accept it, I was relieved. I wasn't alone anymore.

I read articles about the importance of accepting your child's disability. This took a long, long time. Once I came to the realization that this wasn't going away, and that we had to learn to live with her abilities as well as her limitations, I knew I was on my way to acceptance. It was a relief in a way. I didn't reach this level of acceptance easily or quickly. There was no simple way to get to that point. For me, it came after a long period of grieving for the child I expected and hoped to have. Burning that illusion helped me reach some sort of new acceptance.

Since she is so young, it will be years before we know the full extent of the brain injury. Knowing what I know now about what lies ahead, I will have to battle my own prejudice, societal attitudes and chronic sorrow, while fighting battles to help my child reach her full potential.

Healing for families with special needs is a life-long commitment. Every developmental milestone which is not reached brings disappointment and sadness. As my daughter struggles to find her center of balance, our family searches for ours. My healing process began as a quest for knowledge. I read every available resource. But I had a nagging desire to know what the children thought and felt about living with a disability. I wanted to know from adults with special needs how they coped with their disability and what advice they could offer. I needed the insight from family members for support and comfort. And so, the idea for this book was born.

Utilizing my background in psychotherapy, I developed a series of questionnaires for children from the ages of six to eighteen, to be completed, with the assistance of a parent when necessary, for their family members and for adults with disabilities. I also interviewed professionals for advice regarding issues which concern people with disabilities. The issues which were addressed include the following areas: advice, assistance required, communication method, coping skills, discipline, dreams, equipment needed, education experience, fostering independence when possible, heroes, hurdles, leisure activities, motivation, resources, role models, sexuality, spirituality, societal expectations and misconceptions, survival skills and wishes.

The questionnaires were distributed throughout the United States, Ireland and Australia via medical professionals, organizations, newsletters and newspapers. The response was overwhelming. I received letters and telephone calls from all over the country.

This book is a collection of survival stories told by parents, grandparents, children, teenagers and adults who share their honest insight, spirit and determination. My goal in writing this book was not only to provide hope and comfort to families living with special needs, but also to enlighten the public by providing education. Each person in this book is unique. People with disabilities have the same needs as people everywhere. No two people are alike. Their thoughts and feelings are not meant to be representative or generalized to one particular diagnosis or disability.

If someone were to ask me how I would summarize this past year, I guess I would say that I have never cried so hard, been frightened so much and been as vulnerable. When I look back on this past year, I know it has been one of the most exhausting, painful, yet enriching experiences of my life. Through this experience, I was met with kindness and support from most friends, family and professionals. My children have experienced both sorrow and enrichment. They are learning to accept differences and have compassion for others. My husband and I have reached a new level of understanding and patience. I have met people I would have never

Prologue

been able to meet if this had not happened. Of course, I wish this had never happened.

I had the privilege of getting to know families from all over the United States, and a family from Ireland, through their participation in this project. They were willing to share their personal struggles with me. They opened their hearts and souls and for that, I will be forever grateful. They gave me encouragement, support and comfort during my struggle. This knowledge and their survival skills let me know that our family would make it, too. My hope is to provide that same support for others.

Chapter One

THE ROAD TOWARD ACCEPTANCE

The journey toward understanding the implications of the diagnosis is a slow process. Acceptance is unique for each family. Family members feel helpless after being given a diagnosis they know very little about. The information provided may be vague, confusing and overwhelming. The family is in a state of shock. Next, they will be given a treatment plan with a referral for follow-up care in a hospital or an agency. Before they have had time to catch their breath, the parents urgently try to set up their child's next appointment. In the beginning, there is hardly enough time to know what questions need answers. Their sense of desperation and confusion adds to the existing overwhelming grief.

After the family has had some time to acknowledge the impact of the diagnosis, the search for more information begins. The parents want to find honest answers to their questions. For some parents, their child may not have been diagnosed immediately after the parents noticed problems. This may happen because some disabilities are not apparent right away and others do not emerge until the child is older. When this occurs, the parents feel that they have wasted time trying to get the child the appropriate help.

When the family is ready, they begin to piece together the implications of the diagnosis by taking one step at a time. This can be very difficult because the parents may already feel that they have lost time due to a delayed diagnosis. Things move slowly. It takes time to make appointments and receive the necessary services and therapies. It is often a very frustrating period.

Families find that if they are given information about the out-

The Road Toward Acceptance

come of the diagnosis, that gives them a sense of hope, it helps in the midst of their grief. Parents feel less overwhelmed if they are able to make educated decisions for their child's care. This gives them a sense of control over their situation.[2]

Families can regain their sense of balance and decrease helpless feelings when they have answers to questions. Parents become advocates for their child as soon as a diagnosis is given. They advocate to obtain and maintain their child's rights, privileges and services. Parents are better prepared to deal with the needs of their child when they have information about the disability.

Making sense of the diagnosis is the first step toward acceptance. Each family accomplishes this in their own way and in their own time. Parents can request pamphlets or literature from the professional who diagnosed the disability. The information should be easy to read and understand. This information can be copied and given to extended family members or friends who will be involved in the family support network. It helps to give a friend or an extended family member written literature as soon as possible. This helps the parents not to have to answer anymore questions than those for which they are ready.

If literature is not available, parents can ask their physician to write out the specific diagnosis, along with a suggested reading list and resource guide to services. When parents are sitting in the doctor's office listening to the diagnosis, it is often so painful to comprehend, they may not remember what they hear.

When the information is difficult to locate, there are many national and local organizations which provide information free of charge. Direct Link For The Disabled, The Family Resource Center on Disabilities, Mothers United for Moral Support (MUMS), The National Center for Youth with Disabilities and the National Information Clearinghouse for Infants with Disabilities are examples of agencies which serve as information clearinghouses on disabilities. The Resource Guide at the end of this book lists names and addresses of these organizations.

If the child's diagnosis is specific, local or national organizations which deal directly with that disability also can assist with information and referral. United Cerebral Palsy, the National Easter Seal Society, the Mental Health Retardation Authority and the

March of Dimes all provide resource material to families.

Support groups are another way to find resources for the child's care. Other parents can often provide the names of professionals with whom they feel comfortable. The National Parent Network is an example of one such support group. It gives families the name and address of groups in their area. The National Father's Network provides support programs for fathers as well as a quarterly newsletter. The Sibling Information Network has lists of support services and resources for siblings as well as information about starting a sibling support group. The National Self-Advocacy Organization lists self-advocacy groups for people with developmental disabilities throughout the United States.

The family may not have the time nor feel ready to attend support group meetings, but they can always call and request the information they need. Many support groups publish a local resource guide and newsletters which offer advice and practical suggestions.

Once the information search has begun, specific questions which address the child's care can be written down by both parents. The parents can designate one professional with whom they are most comfortable as their care team leader. The professional chosen may be the one who the family feels can provide honest information; the one who helps the family network with other professionals and locate resources. The child's records and reports can be sent to this office, which may serve as a central location to organize the file. As the child's needs change, the care team leader can be the one to request new services and intervention. This person may be the child's neurologist, pediatrician, surgeon or therapist.

An initial meeting with this professional can be set up for both parents to discuss the issues concerning their child. Having the couple participate together in the beginning allows both to become active partners in the child's care. It is often difficult to predict the future for children with disabilities, since so much is unknown. Many parents feel that by remaining hopeful and open regarding the diagnosis, they can survive the unpredictable.

A wide variety of services my be necessary during various stages of the child's development. Building and maintaining a care team depends on locating the correct and most beneficial resources for the family. Services may include medical or surgical interventions, nursing home care, homemaker services, home health aid, hospice care, residential programs, rehabilitation services, nutritional evaluations, educational interventions, therapeutic intervention, such as physical, occupational, speech and respiratory therapy, mental health care and support from counselors, independent living skills, employment training, housing options, and social and recreational opportunities.[3]

To assess which services may be needed for their child, families can request a comprehensive multidisciplinary assessment, which is a team effort to assess the child. They can also choose separate professional assessments which they arrange for privately through a hospital or agency. Both types of assessments will determine the child's strengths and needs. The areas which are reviewed include speech, physical and occupational therapy needs, cognitive skills, learning skills, medical care and health-related issues, vision and hearing screening. The type of assessment and results of the report depend on the developmental age of the child and his or her needs. Such assessments can be found through referrals from the child's physician, a local hospital which serves the needs of children, local organizations which serve specific disabilities, such as United Cerebral Palsy, the local mental health agencies or Early Childhood Intervention Programs (ECI). It may take a long time to uncover all the information. Assessing the initial needs may take weeks and sometimes months. It can take a week or a month to set an appointment and results are not always readily available. The assessments will be repeated over time as the child's needs change.

The family will feel overwhelmed with the results of any testing their child has to go through. They will be spending most of their time learning about a new world. They have to learn about medical techniques such as physical, occupational or speech therapy. The child may require surgeries, medications and procedures about which the family knows very little. They are putting their child's life in the hands of medical professionals they feel anxious about trusting.

During this difficult time, some parents find it helpful to try to simplify their lives. They cancel unimportant outside commitments, ask family members to take care of their other children and have friends take care of some of their basic needs, such as cooking a meal for their family. The family begins to live one day at a time, hour by hour. The most crucial things are the main concern.

First on the list is understanding the diagnosis, then finding the appropriate assessment team and following through with the suggested plan. Their plan may include physical therapy twice a week, occupational therapy twice a week and speech therapy once a week. The family must decide how much therapy they can commit to, remembering that this is only a suggested plan. In the beginning, parents will want to do the most for their child. So, they may follow through by giving their child therapy as often as five days a week. At some point, the parents will want to reevaluate their needs as well as those of their child.

The family always has the option of decreasing or increasing the amount of therapy. They also have the right to seek out the opinions of other professionals regarding treatment options. When parents choose people to work with their child, they should find someone who shares their vision and philosophy for their child. Parents are the ultimate experts on what works best for their child.

Early Childhood Intervention (ECI) Programs

An ECI can provide initial information for families. A referral to an ECI can come from parents, hospitals, physicians, social services or schools. They can be located by contacting each state's Department of Health. They offer services for families who have children from the ages of birth to six and provide interdisciplinary evaluations and intervention services, including physical therapy, education training, self-help skills, parent training, counseling and case management. Linda Horton is the program director for the Early Childhood Intervention Program in Texas. She suggests that families begin with their local ECI to help them learn to cope with the demands of raising a child who has a disability. This program teaches families how to advocate for services and deal with family adjustment issues. Linda recommends that families form a supportive circle of friends, family and professionals. Families experience ambivalent feelings when asking for help.

The Road Toward Acceptance

Learning to trust and rely upon others can help the family adjust.

One Mother Advocates for Services

Elaine Hime is a parent of a six-year-old son who has cerebral palsy and multiple disabilities. She is the founder of the Houston Parent Information Network, a volunteer group which educates families, professionals and the community about the abilities of children with special needs. She started this organization after she searched for resources for her family. She is also a disability specialist for the Parent Education Project with the University of Houston, which serves as an information clearinghouse plus resource center for the community. Elaine has published a potential resource guide for parents of children with disabilities. She recommends finding a pediatrician who has experience treating children with disabilities. The pediatrician she uses for her son, Rutherford, has an understanding of the complex medical issues which affect a child with cerebral palsy. He educates the family and serves as their liaison to the professional community. He organized Rutherford's medical records and helped Elaine's family access programs by helping them understand what labels mean and how to locate services. Certain labels which are attached to the child's diagnosis can benefit the child by qualifying him for various services. Elaine recommends writing down specific names of programs and their locations. At times, there may be confusion finding programs or qualifying financially. Elaine suggests asking to speak to a program supervisor, documenting names and never taking "no" for an answer. When she was trying to qualify for the Women and Infant Care Program (WIC), which provides services for children, including immunizations, milk and formula, she had to advocate for coverage for Rutherford's special nutritional requirements. She qualified for WIC but had to fight to receive it.

Financial Concerns

Once services are found, financial considerations for medical costs create additional pressure. Private insurance policies often cover disability expenses for interventions, such as therapies, equipment, in-home nursing care, nurse-aid service, special formulas and medications. Some policies require letters from physicians stating the necessity of the care. Requirements of individual policy holders depend on each unique policy. If disagreements occur regarding coverage, ask to speak to a supervisor. The family has the right to file a complaint or grievance with their state insurance board.

Medicaid is based on financial need and helps pay for health care for eligible low-income persons. Medicaid applications can be made with each state's department of health or human services. Services covered under Medicaid include hospital care, physician services, eye exams, eyeglasses, ear exams, hearing aids, prescription medication, home health care, early periodic screening, and diagnosis and treatment (EPSDT), which has medical screening and limited dental services to recipients under age 21, transportation services to and from appointments, limited psychiatric service, long-term nursing care and nursing home care, and community facilities for the mentally retarded.[4]

Medicare is available to people who are widowed and have a permanent disability, or workers and people who are over sixty-five years old. It is a federal health program for the aged and people with disabilities. To benefit, one has to have contributed into the federal payroll tax. Social Security Income (SSI) is available to financially needy people who have a disability and the elderly. If a family qualifies for SSI, they can receive Medicaid, housing aid and food stamps.[5] Social Security Disability Insurance (SSDI) is an income maintenance program which people can apply for when they retire, become disabled or upon death of a parent. SSDI is based on work history. Families can contact their local Social Security office for applications and qualifications.

Some hospitals have programs which help families financially by incorporating funds from organizations such as the Lions Club or the Shriners. Families can inquire with the hospital where their child receives care whether they can obtain funding for some for their medical costs through a private charitable organization. There are some nonprofit, private agencies which offer assistance to people who have disabilities. Organizations such as United Cerebral Palsy, the March of Dimes and Muscular Dystrophy offer services. The American Red Cross, the Salvation Army and religious congregations are other resources.

Legal Rights

Families living with disabilities are protected under certain laws and rights. The Americans with Disabilities Act helps people with disabilities to lead more productive lives. The federal government enforces this civil rights legislation. The Americans with Disabilities Act (ADA), Public Law No. 101-336, passed in July of 1990 and is considered to be the true Bill of Rights for people with disabilities. It mandates equal access for people with disabilities to employment, state and local government services, transportation, public accommodations, services provided by private entities and telecommunications. Before the passage of the ADA, discrimination against people with disabilities was only outlawed in certain instances. Section 504 of the Rehabilitation Act of 1973 prohibited discrimination by federally-funded programs only.[6] This law is still in effect.

The Individuals with Disabilities Education Act (IDEA) is a new name for an old law, The Education for All Handicapped Children Act of 1975 Public Law 94-142. This law serves children from ages three to twenty-one. It entitles students with disabilities to receive "free, appropriate education in the least restrictive environment." An individualized education program (IEP) must be assessed to meet each student's learning needs. "Free" education must be provided at no cost in public school. If there is no public school available that can meet the needs of a student, then the public school must pay for the student to attend private school. "Appropriate" means that the needs of each student must be beneficial and decided upon by the family and student. Educational needs which are met must provide the most benefit to the student. "Least restrictive" means students with disabilities are mainstreamed as much as possible with students who are nondisabled. The school must make the necessary accommodations to meet the needs of the students. After age sixteen, the IEP must include a plan for transition to work, college or after graduation.[7]

Public Law 99-457 helps the entire family receive services. This law acknowledges that the family, not just the child with special needs, requires services. This is specifically for children ages birth to two years of age. An individualized Family Service Plan (IFSP) is drafted. Each plan states each service which will be provided. Included in this plan may be siblings needs, parents needs, as well as the needs of child with the disability.

Attitudes

More than forty-three million men, women and children in the United States have a mental or physical disability. These individuals represent approximately one-sixth of the entire population. More than one in every ten people in the country has a special need/disability. The Rehabilitation Act of 1973, Section 504, defines a disability as "any physical or mental impairment that substantially impairs or restricts one or more major life activity; such as caring for one's self, performing manual tasks, walking, seeing, hearing, speaking, breathing, learning or working." The National Organization on Disability (NOD) defines disability as "a permanent physical, sensory or intellectual impairment that substantially limits one or more of a person's major life activities including reading, writing and other aspects of education; holding a job and managing various essential functions of life, such as dressing, bathing and eating." NOD further points out that, "Many of us have disabilities which are visible. Others have disabilities which are invisible. Some disabilities are physical or sensory and others are intellectual or psychological. Some disabilities are temporary, although severely limiting while present. Others are permanent, but need not be fully limiting."[8]

I believe that as a society, we have the moral obligation to create a place where everyone is accepted. Everyone should be entitled to have access to the community, jobs, opportunities, leisure activities and relationships. The first step toward acceptance is knowledge. It is ignorance which leads to fear and prejudice. Changes toward acceptance and disability awareness are occurring throughout the country in areas of employment opportunities, advances in technology, physical fitness activities, travel, media, advertisements, public awareness, educational programs and increased support services for families and individuals with disabilities. Positive steps for change toward inclusion of all people are evolving, but there continues to be attitude barriers.

One mother said, "Attitudes are the real disabilities. There is still a general lack of public knowledge and education which leads to ignorance and prejudice." Attitudes which reflect a lack of education and misinformation regarding people with disabilities increase fear and create prejudice. It is this lack of knowledge which at times separates people and increases feelings of being alone and different. All of the children and teenagers in this book can tell about a time in their lives when they wished someone would have included them rather than have "made fun" of their disability and treated them as "if they were different" when they only longed to be treated "just like everyone else."

A parent of a child who has cerebral palsy and who uses a wheelchair describes an incident which separated her from others. She and her daughter were walking down the street when they saw a mother pull her child closer to her as they walked by, as if they were contagious. The mother of Matthew, an eight-year-old boy who is hearing impaired, feels that as a society, people do not respond well to people with disabilities. She feels that people view them as "dumb or unable to participate in sports." People sometimes stare at her son and say things that are cruel. Arandi's mother feels that society could do a better job responding to those with disabilities. Her twelve-year-old daughter has cerebral palsy and is blind. Some people assume that because Arandi can't see she does not have feelings. Byron, an eleven-year-old boy who has autism, is not accepted by his community. His mother tells of receiving an anonymous letter from a member of their church stating Byron was more "tolerated than accepted." A mother of a six-year-old daughter who has epilepsy feels that people have been both supportive and negative. Sara's mother says that there is very little gray area when it comes to acceptance of her daughter. She finds support from other parents, family members and church. She does not waste her time with those who are negative. She says that by focusing on Sara's medical and educational problems she has become a good advocate for meeting Sara's needs. When she focuses on her entire family, she recognizes how much joy Sara has contributed to their lives. Sara has made her a "better mother, person and friend." Marsha, an eighteen-year-old girl who has cerebral palsy, explains it's important to see people with disabilities as people first. She believes that people with special needs are no different than people who don't have special needs. They just have limitations. Every person with a disability has "different abilities." Randi, a twenty- two-year-old man adds, "Disabled does not mean unable to do."

The goal toward decreasing attitude barriers involves increasing public education, acceptance of diversity, empathy without pity and inclusion and equal participation in community life: jobs, school, housing and relationships.

Suggestions

- Find one organization and request information regarding your child's disability.
- Give information about your child's disability to one extended family member or friend.
- Designate one professional to serve as the care-team leader.
- Start a medical file to organize the child's records.
- Find a local support group and request a newsletter and resource guide.

Chapter Two

THE GRIEVING PROCESS

Strength, patience, joy, pain, love and the capacity to cope are revealed in the face of adversity. The irresistible challenge of life pushes families toward healing and growth. All families meet their needs in different ways. The following true story describes one family's adjustment process.

Mother Blamed for Son's Autism

Joel is a twenty-two-year-old man who has graduated from high school. Though the symptoms appeared when he was twenty-one-months-old, it took two very frustrating years to receive the correct diagnosis of autism. His mother, Becca, says during those years, people were not accustomed to seeing a high-functioning person with autism. Joel was very bright. At twenty-one months, he stopped talking, he stopped looking at people, he would look through them. One month later, he began to print words like "cookie" on paper, and he began to add and subtract numbers on paper with a pencil or on a chalkboard with chalk. Joel was taken to a variety of specialists before the diagnosis was formalized. Becca says it was a nightmare in which she was blamed for Joel's problems. When Joel was a child, autism was thought to be infantile schizophrenia caused by the mother's coldness and inability to bond properly with the child. Mothers were commonly referred to as the "refrigerated mothers." Professionals told her Joel might be mentally retarded, mute, psychotic and have seizures. They told her that they would not treat him until she received counseling. They blamed her. They suggested that she put him away in an institution. It was devastating.

Joel's autism manifested itself through a loss of language; he didn't vocalize or verbalize. Becca became fixated on his loss of language. She thought if he could just talk it would solve everything. He became selectively deaf. He would not hear yelling, but if Sesame Street were on television in the other side of the house, he'd run to the TV. He would avoid eye contact with others. He would look right through them. Joel would take another's hands robotically to reach something to make some kind of contact. He stopped playing with toys. Normal play ceased. He began to play with numbers and letters. He was obsessed with them. He would take dominoes and make math problems with them. He would match up letters and numbers on toy cars. His appetite changed. He stopped eating crunchy food and would only eat mushy food. In social situations, he would walk away from a group. He was on the periphery socially. Becca had to grab him to hug him, which she really needed to do. He had phenomenal fine motor control. At two, he could draw a perfect square.

Becca recalls a repetitive dream about her great desire for Joel to speak to her. He came to her in the dream and spoke the words, "Mama, Mama." One magical morning he did indeed come and speak these words to her. Joel was six and a half. He didn't speak much after that. At age eight, he began to speak a few functional words.

Before this time, he was taught sign language to communicate. He picked this up rather quickly. Becca tells about a funny incident regarding his high intellectual ability. At home Becca and her husband didn't know the correct signs for all the numbers, so to accommodate them, Joel would sign correctly at school and incorrectly at home.

When Joel began to speak, his language was very concrete. He would repeat the ends of phrases and entire sequences said by others. He would become fixated on certain things. For at least one year, he would repeat the entire script of the movie "Annie." He loved public service announcements. He used to repeat "The mind

The Grieving Process

is a terrible thing to waste" and then he'd give out the 800 number. He would say, "The Peace Corps, the toughest job you'll ever love."

His favorite television show remains Wall Street Week. He repeats lines that moderator Lewis Ruykeiser says. He has even dressed for Halloween like Lewis Ruykeiser. When Joel was practicing for his bar mitzvah, he repeated lines from Wall Street Week. He started by saying, "Good evening ladies and gentlemen, I'm Lewis Ruykeiser." The rabbi just bowed his head and said, "Becca, I see what you mean."

Joel's educational experience began poorly. He attended a developmental preschool. His family requested a hearing at Joel's next school because the administration would not create an appropriate class for him. Three days before the case was to be heard in federal court, the school board created a communication disorders class. One week later, sixteen children were enrolled. After one year, Joel's needs were not being met, so he attended a mental health center which only met his behavioral needs, not language needs. His third school was a special education school twenty-three miles from their home. The school would not transport Joel by bus, so Becca had to drive every day. She describes it as a horrible self-contained classroom with a teacher who worked a lot on behavior and little on anything else. Twelve years ago, the family moved to Phoenix and into a new, very good school. Joel had five productive years there. The staff used a combination of techniques which Becca found very helpful and effective. They used firm behavior management, direct language instruction—which Becca referred to as "in your face speech therapy"—and a variety of ways to get a child to communicate. They didn't let him withdraw. The assumption of the teachers was that each child/student would succeed. They taught fine arts, dance, creative movement and adaptive physical education. They had a high-energy staff. The school got Joel to initiate conversation and he is able now to communicate his needs.

In high school, Joel was partially mainstreamed. Becca says there were very positive elements. They met a lot of people who cared and Joel had a regular math teacher who took him all the way up to pre-calculus. This teacher used love, patience, affection and good nature.

Becca says she advises parents to go into their child's school experience with a positive attitude and not assume the school is the enemy. They need to do their homework before the child begins school and learn the laws which apply to the school. Documenting the child's performance and knowing his or her current level of functioning is important. Bringing all documentation to meetings is a must. Don't be afraid to set challenging goals which have meaning. Make sure the Individualized Education Program includes behavior, social self-help, recreation and academic goals. Find out what the school will do to meet each goal and ask for specifics.

Becca described her family as a "typical all-American family, wonderful and proud. My husband and I have been married for twenty-four years. They have been twenty-four challenging, stressful years with remarkable blessings and achievements."

She started the Council for Jews with Special Needs, which serves children and adults with disabilities. Joel is employed at the county library part-time and his job involves sorting and shelving, which require accuracy and perfection. "What better job for someone like Joel. It took awhile for the librarians and support staff to become comfortable with Joel."

The staff asked Becca for the titles of books on autism and read up on the subject. Joel tends to talk out loud and sing to himself while he works. One day the staff working near him began to sing along with him. Joel stopped sorting and stared at his co-workers as they sang to him. When they finished, he said, "You did that very well."

Learning to Cope With Grief

Chronic sorrow is a term often used to describe the whirlwind of emotions felt by family members adjusting to disabilities throughout lifetime milestones, reached or not reached. After the initial shock wears off, the road to acceptance is long and difficult. Recycling through the grieving process takes place for the entire family and may be experienced at different times.

There is no typical pattern of grieving. Everyone grieves in

The Grieving Process

their own way in their own time. The stages of grief are described as denial, anger, bargaining, depression and eventual acceptance. The stages are referred to as tasks: alarm and shock, searching, mitigation or freedom from pain, anger and guilt, recovery.[9] The phases or tasks do not occur in a sequential order. They may occur in the course of five minutes or over a period of days, months or years.

During the initial phase, parents often feel terrified. They are in a state of shock. After a diagnosis is confirmed, there is often the hope that it is a mistake. They wonder if they will be able to manage the overwhelming responsibilities which come with taking care of a child with a disability. Depression, feelings of weariness and numbness are often felt due to the physical and mental exhaustion which occur in the face of new demands. Sleep disturbance either in the form of insomnia or wanting too much sleep is common during this phase. Loss of appetite, overeating, restlessness, irritability and decreased sexual drive can occur.[10]

Parents feel as if they are falling apart. Social isolation adds to the growing despair. Friends and family may be unable to provide support due to their uncomfortable feelings. They may feel helpless and not know what to do for the family. Some stay away. The family has new demands placed upon them. They are learning how to cope in the midst of emotional and physical exhaustion. Explanations to friends and family become increasingly difficult. Questions from others cannot be readily answered. The time once spent on other activities is replaced with medical appointments and new responsibilities. The time left over for anyone else is limited.

Feelings of anger and guilt often accompany the search for answers. At times, anger is directed at caregivers, family, friends, God, themselves, the unjust situation and at the child with the disability.[11] Families want to know what caused the disability and the future implications. They often ask what could have been done to prevent the situation. Parents feel as if they have not done enough. Family members feel as if they have lost control of their lives and resent the new demands. The parents feel guilty because they feel angry toward those around them.

Parents often look for a way out of the situation. As their feelings fluctuate, they bargain and look for cures. They wish they were the ones who had the disability. They feel despair and frustration because they cannot fix the situation. They feel as if they have failed their child in some way. They protest the situation and deny the reality so as to avoid the painful feelings. It is during this time that the family is trying to make sense of what has happened. They try to come to terms with the disability. They wish to mitigate the pain.[12] The family searches for ways to make life bearable and they grieve the dream of the child that they had hoped to have while beginning to come to terms with the child they do have.

Gradually, on their own and within their own time frame, the family accepts the situation. They recover and discover a new identity for themselves.[13] They slowly move back into a routine of daily living. New relationships, different activities and new patterns begin to form. Old relationships are redefined. Acceptance should not be mistaken for forgetting. Acceptance means that one comes to the realization that they have experienced a great loss, and that never goes away. Acceptance occurs as one learns to adjust to a new lifestyle with the changes that require setting a new pace and learning new tasks. This is often a vulnerable time for families as they learn to test the water. They may feel ready to go out socially with old friends only to feel overwhelmed by the situation and want to return home.

Sorrow resurfaces in varying degrees and levels of intensity as families cross new hurdles, delays and disappointments in the child's progress or lack of progress. Missed or delayed milestones, holidays and special occasions serve as landmarks and can trigger feelings of grief. Sorrow can crop up at the most unexpected moments—a look or comment from a stranger inquiring about the disability or seeing a new baby in the grocery store. Going to the child's physical therapy appointment and watching a child with a disability struggle to play with a toy and going to a family get-together and watching children without disabilities play can trigger profound emotions. These unexpected moments catch parents off-guard. They may find themselves feeling sad and crying. This is part of grieving as well. These daily events remind parents of the reality of their situation. They are grieving for their ideal child and are reminded that their child will have to struggle for those things that other children will take for granted. It is a long and slow process to release the illusion of the child the family had expected to have and accept the child they do have. It is not a process to be rushed.

A Mother's Story of Sorrow

Barbara is a mother of a twenty-one-year-old son who has Down Syndrome. Even though she feels that life is full of "wonders" and can see this in her son, she struggles with her feelings. Her son, Steve, lives at home and works in a sheltered workshop. Steve's verbal ability is limited due to a high palate, but he is able to communicate by using sign language. It is a tough road for their family. They find people to be uncaring. The amount of paperwork and red-tape they have to go through to arrange services for Steve is overwhelming. At times, Barbara struggles with her own fears and doubts about the amount of independence she should give her son. She has encouraged Steve to go places in a cab, alone, but is always uncertain about her decision to trust a complete stranger to drive her son. Barbara knows that Steve is not the easiest person to live with. He fights going to work and is rather lazy and immature. It is sometimes hard for Barbara to have patience. When Steve expresses that he would someday like to marry and have a home of his own, it breaks Barbara's heart because she feels that this is impossible for her son.

If feelings of grief become consistently more difficult to deal with and interfere with daily living, professional counseling can help family members learn coping skills. Dr. Kenneth Kopel is a clinical psychologist and clinical faculty member with Baylor University. He specializes in helping families cope with chronic medical issues. He encourages those who are grieving to give themselves permission to talk about their feelings with an empathic person or to join a support group. They should know that their feelings, as intense as they may be at times, are normal and real. The duration of grieving varies. It is okay to not feel the way society or other people expect you to feel. Friends or family may say things that seem horrifying or hurtful. This is not to imply that they are cruel; often they do not realize how they sound. Be aware of this. Some people may withdraw due to their own uncomfortable feelings or inability to feel helpful. This does not mean those who cannot be supportive are good or bad people. It helps to redefine old relationships and know that only some people will be there for the family and others may withdraw and return later or not at all. Finding new avenues of support helps the family decrease the sense of isolation. Eventually, there is a very slow and subtle process which occurs when one learns to cope. Families learn to get past the intense grief and move on to a different level. There seems to be a natural adjustment whereby one awakens and does not feel the heavy, deep depression. To reach this point, Dr. Kopel suggests, "parents put on their oxygen mask first to catch their breath and then take care of the children." Recharging themselves by taking time out alone and with their partner enables them to renew their ability to carry on at home. It is okay to go out and enjoy time without the children without feeling guilty. How well the family survives depends on the coping skills they had before the diagnosis when handling crises and the ability to incorporate these skills into the existing situation. To move on, parents need an attitude of accepting themselves, not trying to be perfect and knowing that the family will survive. The following is a true story from a mother who is learning to cope with the demands that come with raising a seven-year-old daughter who has multiple birth defects and anomalies.

A Mother's Story

Autumn's mother describes her daughter as being of average height and weight, with dark brown hair, china-doll white skin, big blue eyes and a surgery scar from nose to lip. Autumn is very strong-willed. She gives the best hugs in the world, and lots of them, is joyous to a fault and doesn't care who catches it from her. She can turn tears on and off at the speed of light. When she was very young, she slept with her books, videos and software boxes. She has no concept of evil, which is worrisome to her mother. She fakes headaches and stomachaches to get out of math at school or "yukky" supper or homework. Autumn loves to collect things:

pictures, cards, little Disney characters. Their house usually looks like they have twelve children instead of one. Autumn has some unique habits that intrigue the family. She had lots of paperback Disney books and matching cassette tapes, but she became bored with each book, so somehow she disassembled all of them. Now she has two or three hundred individual pages, and they are like gold to her. She arranges and rearranges them in various formations. They look like random samplings, but if anyone tampers with even one pile, she becomes upset. It seems so peculiar, but Autumn's parents decided to trust her; she might be organizing some brain activity or something. Being Autumn's parent is like having a second full-time job, so leisure doesn't come often. The three do enjoy each other's company, going out to eat, to the malls, sometimes to the movies, once in a while to a play or the circus. They are very involved in the activities of their church.

Although the only obvious problem at birth was a cleft lip and palate, as time went by, more and more of Autumn's multiple birth defects and anomalies surfaced. Her mother calls it the Autumn Theorem: If you take Autumn to a specialist, they will find something wrong.

To date, we know: in all of her cells, Autumn has an extra piece of her thirteenth chromosome (Trisomy 13), and in thirty percent of her cells, she has another smaller piece, possibly from the eleventh or seventeenth chromosome. She has partial agenesis of the corpus callosum, ACC, the large bundle of nerves connecting the two hemispheres of her brain. This was discovered in a CAT scan done when Autumn was about three or four months old. At the time, few conclusions were drawn and the family was so involved in surgeries for the cleft lip and palate, and her eyes, no one realized the full significance of the CAT scan. Only very recently have they become aware that probably all of Autumn's difficulties are the result of this one aspect.

The cleft lip and palate are a midline birth defect occurring in many children with ACC, and many without. Cosmetically speaking, surgery fixed Autumn up beautifully. She simply has a small scar from her nose to her lip. Her palate was repaired surgically, affecting her speech, however Autumn has never been able to speak intelligibly, or much at all, as a result of ACC. In all, she's had five surgeries relating to this. Still to come is a bone graft within her gumline and probably some cosmetic surgery on her nose. A condition called strabismus affected Autumn's eyes and they did not focus together until it was corrected by two surgeries. Her big, beautiful eyes work together well now; however, she is a little farsighted and wears glasses. Autumn has a much greater problem, however, in that all her motor abilities—speech being a very complex motor ability—are affected by the neurological involvement of the ACC. Her speech and motor planning are affected, causing motor dyspraxia. In lay terms, this means that when she encounters a new task of some sort, her nervous system doesn't give her adequate information to accomplish it. She has a general developmental delay. She didn't walk until twenty-one months, has never been able to pedal a tricycle or bicycle, cannot grip tight enough to write or draw. She jumped for the first time at about age four, but she doesn't have the kind of light bounciness needed for continual rope jumping. She has been trying to skip for several years but doesn't quite have it down yet. Her lower body is very sturdy and strong, but her upper body has low muscle tone and she's as weak as a kitten. Last summer, she had six weeks of swimming lessons and it seems to have benefited her in every way: strength, coordination, muscle tone, self-confidence. Plans call for more swimming lessons. She has not needed adaptive physical education at school and her physical education teachers say she's doing well and making progress. When she was four, the family bought a computer and it was as if they'd found one of the keys to unlock Autumn. She learned the keyboard very quickly and is able to move in and out of different games and software applications after being shown just once. She generally uses only her thumbs and forefingers, but occasionally she is caught trying her elbows, nose and chin! Next, the family purchased an augmentative communication device, a DigiVox, which is a computer and tape-recorder combination. It's limited in that she can only say what it is programed to say, but it has been extremely helpful in the classroom, allowing Autumn to participate in class discussions and out-loud reading. Each Friday, her teacher sends home the next week's lessons, and her parents program it all onto "the box," as it's affectionately called. A family friend, a juvenile-sounding fifteen-year-old, supplies Autumn's voice on the box. Autumn is enthused about using this device only as long as the information on it stays new and updated. She gets private speech therapy and occupational therapy at school and for the past three years has had sensory integration therapy from a private therapist.

Autumn attends regular first grade. She leaves the classroom for thirty minutes each day to get some one-on-one help. While the rest of the class draws and writes about their lives, Autumn scans pictures onto a computer screen and types her sentences below. Beyond that, she is totally included in all activities with her peers. Her teacher assures me the curriculum has not been modified for Autumn. She is not required, however, to generate the volume of work, as her hands work more slowly than those of her peers. She also needs help focusing and concentrating, and is quite easily distracted. This is true at home as well. She has difficulty following through on tasks independently. Autumn is included in every way with her nondisabled peers and she is learning normal social interaction. She will gradually learn her limits and will have to accept them and adjust her goals accordingly, as we all do. The technology in the public school has benefited her in every way, and she could not get an education without it. At this point, school is totally affirming for Autumn. She is very well known and her self-esteem is very high. She really loves school and learning, and she needs structure and discipline. Her teachers are all hopelessly bonded to her for life.

Autumn's mother finds taking it one day at a time most difficult. She says she often projects into the future and it can be very frightening. She's learning, however, that she wastes a lot of perfectly good worry doing that, because most of her worries never come to pass. She agrees with a saying she heard recently, "Worry is just a mental gimmick we use to give us the illusion that we can control the future." One of the things most tempting for her to worry about is that Autumn will not have a social life as she gets older because of her inability to speak and her developmental delay. She is very innocent, less sophisticated than other children her age. She isn't as aware of cultural standards or of what society expects of people. She's more like a younger child in some ways and very vulnerable.

In Autumn's mother's words: "I see a real conflict within myself about her independence. On the one hand, I recognize that I have a really intense emotional need for her to look cute or perform correctly or to 'fit in,' so I have to work hard at making myself let her decide things: what to wear, what to buy, what to eat, who to play with. I desperately don't want her to be weird, to be an outcast, because that would be so painful to me. I recognize that this is my problem, not hers, and I don't hesitate to get counseling when I need it. I want to be free to accept her for who she is, not force her to be what I need her to be. On the other hand, I get discouraged sometimes when she insists on being babyish and dependent, or when she truly cannot do something by herself, like putting on her socks or entertaining herself. A friend of mine said, 'She may always need help putting her socks on, but you must empower her within herself.' I'm not sure how to do that, but I intend to learn. One day she'll turn around and tell us to get a life, and then I'll know we did okay. As far as encouraging my own independence, I think it's very important, if time and energy permit, to maintain some interests apart from her, something that develops me as a person. Then, on the day she tells me to get a life, I'll be able to say, 'I've got one, ha ha!' She's only seven, and I know much harder days are coming on this subject. So ask me this question in seven more years. I often just grit my teeth and look the other way while she struggles. I keep reminding myself that if I keep her dependent on me, there will come a day when she'll resent me for it. So I keep working on it. Right now the goals are all pretty short-term. We have a chart on the refrigerator listing a few duties and each time she does one, she gets a star. It has kind of evolved over the past couple of years. The three things on the chart currently are household chores: making her bed, setting the table and feeding the cat. When she gets twenty-five stars, we go on a shopping trip and she can get anything she wants (not to worry, her tastes lean toward the simple). We're currently discussing doing away with the chart, instituting the chores as just part of life with no reward, and giving her an allowance.

"Autumn has gone through some stages of being really defiant, but mostly she's a pretty complaint-free little kid. She's very loving and can't stand for a relationship to be broken for long. We borrowed a video from our speech therapist about a simple method of counting. When behavior starts to get out of hand, we say, 'That's 1,' If it continues, 'That's 2.' If we get to 3, she 'Takes 5,' which means five minutes alone in her room; hell on earth for Autumn. Autumn can test our patience almost to the breaking point because she has difficulty finishing even a simple task. She gets her underwear up to her knees and is off doing something else, or her toothbrush makes it into her mouth but never moves once it's there. That used to make for a lot of eye-rolling and even yelling on my part, especially when getting ready for school and work every morning. But the video talked about setting a kitchen timer while the task gets done and Autumn's been really responsive to that. The penalty for not getting the task finished before the bell rings is usually no TV. She hustles! Although we knew about the corpus callosum years ago, we recently did some new reading on it and discovered that much of the stuff that tests our patience is probably not done to intentionally drive us crazy, but because she has difficulty concentrating. So the new knowledge has helped us be more patient.

"Autumn's only beginning to be aware of her differences; there will be more to relate to in the future. We are only beginning to discuss this with her. Only this past year has she seemed to notice the scar on her lip. So I showed her pictures of how she looked after various surgeries, and she seems content with that. Also, this year I've taken the bull by the horns and asked her if it makes her sad that all her friends can talk, skip or ride a bike, and she can't. She said yes, and so in very simple words, I explained that when she was growing inside me, something in her brain didn't grow exactly right, and that makes it harder for her to learn some things. We've had the same discussion two or three times, and she seems to accept it readily. She doesn't use words to describe her disability to others. Her friends usually address their questions about that to me, and I say generally the same things to them but on a lighter note. I don't believe that Autumn has fully grasped her own situation yet. She went to an excellent preschool for children with special needs, and we've maintained friendships with one or two families. But we see them infrequently and their needs are pretty different from Autumn's. She prefers her non-disabled friends."

Open your heart to the fact that our children are gifts to us, not crosses to bear. And I don't mean that God gives special children to special people. We aren't special. If that's what special means, let me be mediocre!

Autumn's Mother Reflects

"Having Autumn constantly confronts me with my own prejudices and fears, and it forces me to deal with them and grow past them. It forces me to examine my ideas of human worth, including my own. It forces me to confront my limits; I have to keep coming again and again to the realization that this is too big for me, that I can't fix Autumn, that sometimes I can't even cope with all this. And somehow in the process I have gotten to know God in such a deep, personal way, and I know now absolutely that he loves me and Autumn and all of us more than we can imagine. It is living with her and observing how he champions her cause that has won my heart over to him. So that personal knowledge is in itself a very great gift. I would advise parents to network with other families of kids with special needs, and with professionals in the field. Stay up to date and informed about your child's disabilities. And don't accept someone else's limitations and predictions about your child! Love is a powerful healer.

"One of the most common misconceptions regarding disabilities is that doctors, educators, professionals, as well as myself, believe that developmental delays are static, fixed, all-pervasive and eternal. We have all had the good fortune to be in contact with many others who scoff at that notion. Early intervention with various therapies and the right kind of education can open all kinds of possibilities.

"I think there's hope for the next generation, and even my own! My experience has been that none of my fears about 'society' have become a reality so far. In our case anyway, Autumn is met everywhere with smiles, compassion, interest and friendship. This tells me that things are looking up, that Autumn's generation could be truly different from my own. And this is the result of more and more inclusion of disabled people into the mainstream at an age when children are just forming their world view."

The Grieving Process

Acceptance

Holding children or adults with disabilities to a different standard of living creates unrealistic pressure for them as well as their families. Just as parents do not want to be considered "courageous" or "saints," neither do their children. Nor do people want to be underestimated for their abilities. Broad generalizations which overestimate or underestimate one's potential only contribute to stereotyping and prejudice. A mother of an eight-year-old girl, Danielle, who has cerebral palsy, often hears people say, "Oh, you're a saint," or "What special people you are." Her reply is, "No, we're not. We love her and choose to take responsibility for her well-being."

Becca, Joel's mother, suggests that people should not define anyone by the disability. There is an assumption that people with special needs have an inferior quality or should have superachieving qualities. They are people first, with many abilities.

Barbara, a thirty-two-year-old woman who is deaf, suggests that parents accept what their children choose. "Don't try to make them into something they are not. Accept the disability and don't try to change them."

The mother of Siobhan, an eleven-year-old girl who was born with a chromosome disorder that causes severe mental, physical and developmental retardation, stresses the importance of acceptance. She feels that her family is ordinary and has not been chosen by God because he knew that they would be able to look after a "special" child. It took years for Siobhan's mother to come to terms with her child's disability. She felt that by giving herself time to grieve and sharing practical advice and feelings with other parents who have children with disabilities helped her accept Siobhan for who she is.

Suggestions

- Understand that coming to terms with loss takes time and does not follow any pattern.
- Find one person to share thoughts and feelings with to de-

crease a sense of isolation. Form a support circle of friends, family, clergy and parents who have children with disabilities.

- Fulfill your own needs by taking time alone and with your spouse to recharge without feeling guilty.
- Accept your own limitations and those of your children.
- It is okay to not feel the way others expect you to feel. Our feelings, as intense as they may be, are normal and real.

Chapter Three

THE MARRIAGE

Marital stress is an inevitable part of life. Family dynamics change over time due to economic stress, children's behavior, discipline or sibling problems, insufficient couple time, lack of shared responsibility in the family, communication difficulties, insufficient personal time, guilt for not accomplishing more, intimacy problems, insufficient family playtime and an overscheduled family calendar.[14] The marriage in a special needs family has to face the normal strain plus the added pressures of living with and taking care of a child who has a disability. They also are living with physical and emotional exhaustion, which exacerbates everything. The couple has to summon up the energy to call on old coping skills while trying to piece together a treatment plan for their child and grieve a loss. The ability to deal effectively with stress is related to how much prior experience the couple has had in coping with strain.[15]

Couples who survive tragedies have certain characteristics which enable them to rise above the stress and re-establish their relationship.[16] They utilize support systems for strength. They view calling upon family, friends, spiritual guidance, counseling or support groups as a positive step to help them understand the magnitude of their loss. They learn to transcend their guilt and regrets. They refuse to be bitter and replace this with a sense of hope regarding the future. They discuss their feelings openly with one another but give each other room to breathe, respecting each other's habits and needs. They creatively manage conflicts by problem-solving and defining issues that need resolution. The couple learns to distinguish between those events they can and cannot control. They focus on those they can control and develop workable ways of solving problems, which requires communication and perseverance. The couple is adaptable; they borrow each other's skills and resources.

They each grieve in different ways and during different times. Rutherford's father seemed to accept his son's cerebral palsy right away. Rutherford's mother, Elaine, said people misinterpreted her husband's quick acceptance as denial. Other parents describe feeling solely responsible for their child's care. Byron's mother feels as though she is raising her twelve-year-old son alone. It has become a full-time job. Her marriage has suffered under the strain. She recommends that parents be equally responsible for the care of the child with the disability. Otherwise, one takes on too much. Byron's mother believes that both parents should take an active role in planning the child's future. They should support each other emotionally to decrease isolation and stress.

Each partner in the marriage copes in different ways. They each experience a myriad of feelings. The fear of expressing painful feelings sometimes holds one partner back from sharing his true reactions. Feelings of guilt, realistic or unrealistic, surface. Feeling guilty may overwhelm the parent to the point where they avoid the child. Parents may have resentful feelings and then feel ashamed for feeling that way.

Problem Solving

Dr. Ken Kopel, a clinical psychologist, suggests that couples share their painful emotions and redefine their roles within the marriage. This allows the couple to validate their feelings. Parents may not feel the same things at the same times. Respecting that each person has different feelings is important. He recommends that each partner discuss how they can divide duties and responsibilities so that one partner does not take over too much. The couple calls upon their own resources and decides upon a workable plan. The partners decide what issues need resolving and determine which events they can control. An example may be dividing responsibilities for the children in the family.

The Marriage

Each person decides which tasks or parts of tasks they feel comfortable doing. For instance, one partner may feel most comfortable taking their child with the disability to medical appointments and the other may take over the daily home care such as dressing, bathing and feeding. Another task which can be divided or taken on by one spouse may be taking care of the medical files. One may look for potential resource material for the family: support groups, information related to the disability, formulating a treatment plan for the child. Taking care of the other children in the family is yet another task which can be shared.

The couple should discuss ways they can take breaks together and alone. This enables each partner to have private time and meet his needs. It may be beneficial to locate respite care or a sitter who can relieve the parents, so they can have time together. Sharing feelings, creating a workable plan after defining issues, and taking time away can help couples live with a chronic situation.

A Father's Story

Here a father tells of his feelings of frustration as he attempts to deal with his daughter's disability.

"I had just ordered a bottle of our favorite wine when my wife was brought over to the table by the maitre d'. In his always pleasant manner, he began pointing out several modifications to the menu that had been made since we last ate at our favorite restaurant.

"No one had seen us out socially since we learned that our youngest daughter had been diagnosed with cerebral palsy. In the last several months, my wife had read every medical book, article and resource available to educate herself while I immersed myself further in my work. My colleagues, who knew, acted like nothing was wrong. Life went on.

"I had no reference point. I wasn't the one going to play group or being asked why my daughter wasn't walking. It made it easier for me to pretend that a few physical therapy sessions would loosen up her ankle.

"Ironically, as a personal injury lawyer, I deal with injury and people's suffering on a daily basis. In fact, embellishing on the suffering of my clients is what my legal experience has taught me maximizes jury verdicts.

"This, however, was an injury far too close to home; one that was initially unacceptable, but as my wife explained, had to be confronted.

"Soon the getaway evening I had planned had turned into a lesson in reality. My wife informed me the physical therapist thinks that our daughter might get around better with the help of a walker. My heart sank; after all, walkers are for disabled people, not my child. Little did I know that dealing with her condition had several such reality checks over the months that followed.

"With the brace changes, injections of Botox, a muscle relaxer, doctor visits, therapies and the agonizing unknown, I look at the face of our beautiful, smiling two-year-old, innocent and unaware that she suffers from any limitations. In fact, that walker we discussed was never purchased, and soon after she began walking. Although I know that with time other problems, such as her current inability to speak, the unbelievable lack of understanding, and lack of resources available, will in all likelihood continue to surface, I stand committed to face those realities."

Dealing with Isolation

Often the family is too exhausted and lacks the time to be with others. Everything takes longer: feeding, dressing, communicating. It becomes difficult to deal with strangers, family and friends' comments, stares and advice. Well-meaning outsiders often say things out of ignorance or curiosity due to a lack of education regarding disabilities. Going to the grocery store becomes a challenge. Parents are often torn between explaining the child's disability for education sake and not wanting to be bothered by others. Isolation replaces socialization.

Psychotherapist Terry Phillips Whitman helps people cope with chronic medical issues. She suggests some ways couples can deal with loss. Often, couples who face chronic situations become isolated because they feel that others do not understand their pain. When this occurs, friends, family and the other spouse are pushed away. People who are grieving are frightened because they feel alone in their pain and then feel helpless to do anything about their intense feelings. Painful feelings are very difficult for others to face and they feel helpless because they cannot fix the situation or make the person better. They are uncomfortable with the intensity of the emotions and sometimes withdraw. The person in pain feels like a burden to others and then pulls away further. De-isolation for the person who is in the most pain is important. Sharing painful feelings and understanding the magnitude of the loss helps people move beyond the pain. This can be accomplished by finding a support group with people who are in a similar situation or an empathic person who will listen.

Sharing feelings and experience helps to validate feelings and decrease isolation. People who share a common bond do not feel so burdened by the intense feelings the situation brings about. The more supported a person feels, the less likely he or she will feel like a burden on others. Eventually, relationships, activities and daily living will take place outside of the painful experience.

By letting others know that they are not responsible for making you feel happy or take away your sadness, the burden is lifted. Telling your spouse, "Let me be sad, allow me to cry and stay with me," allows for supportive grieving and validation of feelings. But, there is a need to be understood and feel the same things together, and when one partner does not feel the same way it brings about anger and frustration. This difference in expression is a natural part of grieving a loss. It helps if each partner allows the other to feel the way they need to, and to accept that. One spouse may say, "I feel lonely because you don't feel the same way." The partners can reassure each other that it is okay to have different feelings.

Starting a support group

If a support group is not available to meet the needs of the parents, they can start one. Eve Cugini is the director of Family to Family Network, a support group that serves over 500 families in Texas. It is a local grass-roots organization made up of families and friends of children with disabilities. They work together to create a community where all children belong. Eve started Family to Family during her search for resources for her five-year-old son who has cerebral palsy. There are many benefits to meeting other families in a similar situation. After a diagnosis has been established, the family needs a safe place to vent feelings without having to explain. Families share concrete, honest and practical information with each other which can be a source of strength. Parents who use support groups define their own needs and what they expect to gain from the experience. Everyone comes to the group at different points, with different feelings and varied experiences.

Eve suggests some guidelines to start a support group if there is not one available. A mission statement which defines the shared vision of the group should be established early on and may change as the needs of the group change. The statement should include who will be involved in the group as well as the purpose. Family to Family defines itself as a grass-roots organization made up of families and friends of children with disabilities. Its purpose is to work together to create a community where all children belong.

The purpose of the group is defined by short- and long-term goals. Short-term goals include how often meetings will be held and where, and what information will be conveyed at meetings. Information may include advice on things like juggling schedules, identifying resources, or how to advocate for services from therapists or the school system. Informal gatherings which are social in nature, such as picnics and potluck suppers, are a good way to get families together in a fun atmosphere. Formal sharing may involve inviting a professional from the community to discuss issues concerning families with disabilities. A lawyer who specializes in future planning with families could discuss practical ways to ensure that parents are preparing for their child's future. The group may want to include a mentorship program. They can invite adults with disabilities to share information with families about growing up with special needs. The adults can serve as role models to the children as well as the parent.

Long-term goals include the future dreams of the group, such

The Marriage

as establishing a lending library for families, having members attend educational seminars, having parents take training courses on advocacy or establishing a teen network that provides support and activities.

A newsletter can be a very useful information resource. It serves as a lifeline to those members who do not have time to attend meetings. Parents share information through various columns. Features can include news and happenings on the state and federal front, school success stories, family profiles, resource section, legislative updates, conferences, activities and information, and parent requests for equipment through want ads.

The group may want to set up committees for outreach, fundraising, public relations and social activities. Officers can be selected to be on the board of directors. A president, vice president, secretary and treasurer can be chosen to represent the group. Applying for nonprofit status to become known as a charitable organization is beneficial. A 501 C 3 application can be requested from the Secretary of State's office.

New members can be solicited in a variety of ways. There are a number of existing family support groups, such as Mothers United for Moral Support, which hooks up families with similar disabilities and rare medical conditions. The National Father's Network and the National Parent Network, may be starting places to look for families. They have newsletters which can advertise a new support group (see Resource Guide).

The American Self-Help Clearinghouse will provide current information and contacts for any national self-help groups that deal with specific disabilities. It also provides The Self-Sourcebook, which contains ideas for starting a support group, as well as contacts for more than 600 national and model groups.

Many families find support through their local religious congregation. Some families have gained strength through their spiritual belief. Members of their churches and synagogues provide support by offering to babysit to give the couple a break, as well as cooking meals for the family. Rabbis, priests and ministers provide a source of comfort by listening to the concerns of all family members.

The National Organization of Disability (NOD) has developed

the Religion and Disability Program, which assists churches and synagogues in becoming more sensitive. They have two booklets which explain specific ways congregations can open their doors for people who have disabilities, "Loving Justice" and "That All May Worship".

Suggestions

- Share feelings with each other and understand the magnitude of the loss.
- Join a support group for families with children who have disabilities or find one family who shares a common bond. This provides a sense of hope that others can transcend their loss.
- Respect each other's needs and habits. Take breaks together and apart. Find a sitter or respite care worker who can help with the children to give you a chance to go out.
- Define issues which need resolution and devise a workable plan, which includes dividing and sharing tasks and responsibilities.
- Focus on those things which can be controlled and on finding information related to the disability which will help the family.

Chapter Four

THE SIBLINGS

Sisters and brothers adjust best to having a sibling with a disability when feelings, thoughts and concerns are expressed and communicated in an honest and open manner. The other children in the family usually reflect the same emotions and thoughts as their parents.[17] Parents have a very influential position in helping other family members adjust to their new roles, responsibilities and feelings. Balancing all the children's needs in the family with unconditional love and acceptance helps to increase everyone's self-esteem.

It was once assumed that families were incapable of taking care of a child with a special need without neglecting the care of the other children. The siblings were thought to suffer from more psychological problems than "normal siblings in normal families."[18] They were thought to be neglected, abused and given more responsibilities than other children. Some of these assumptions came about due to stereotyping and the stigma attached to raising a child with a special need. Children do experience feelings and reactions about their brother or sister's special needs. They show concern just as any brother or sister does for any sibling. These feelings do not mean that later they will develop behavioral disorders or psychological problems.

Children and youth in special needs families experience the same feelings about their siblings as all children do, but there are some feelings common to children with siblings who have special needs. They can be summarized by age range.[19] Not all children experience these feelings or reactions, however.

Preschool children fear being separated from their parents. If the parents must spend excessive amounts of time taking the sibling to the doctor, hospital or to other special appointments, the child at home will become frightened, and may feel left out and unloved. He may feel jealous of and angry toward the other child. Parents may find that this child has excessive tantrums, exhibits unusual behavior and develops sleeping problems. The child may regress, withdraw or try to please to attempt to get attention. The parents need to spend more one-on-one time by playing a game he enjoys or doing a household chore together. This private time together can help reassure the child that there is still positive routine in their lives. To help children deal with their feelings, parents can support and validate their struggle. Giving them opportunities to express themselves, to come to an understanding and make some meaning out of difficult situations is important. Children will feel most comfortable when family problems are discussed. Parents can help preschool children release their feelings through art projects such as drawing and painting. Younger children are not always able to find the words to express their feelings, but they may show them with crayons, paint, paper and dolls. Parents can reassure their children and decrease fears of separation by holding and comforting and talking.

Keeping a routine in family life helps children go on with daily living. The mother and father can ask all the children in the family to help with responsibilities around the house. Each child can be assigned age-appropriate chores. Making the beds, feeding the pets and hanging up their clothes are examples of ways to ensure that everyone pitches in. When appropriate, it is okay to involve brothers and sisters in their sibling's therapy. The children can be brought along to therapy sessions and can help out by rolling a ball or getting a toy. This will make them feel part of the process and decrease any sense of mystery. At the same time, it will decrease some fears of separation.

A school-age sibling will be concerned with what his friends think about the disability. They may not want to bring their school friends home because they are embarrassed by how the child with special needs will appear to the friend. The child may experience conflicting feelings regarding his sibling. He may feel that he has

The Siblings

to perform and excel to make up for the other child. He may feel embarrassed and horrified because of the appearance or behavior of the sibling. He may worry that somehow the condition of the sibling was caused by something he wished for or said. Another common feeling is guilt, related to feeling resentful toward the child with the special need because of the extra time parents spend with him. Sometimes, the child may worry excessively about the sibling and he may hover over him. Parents can reassure the sibling by giving him supportive information about the disability to alleviate the fear of the unknown, which may be behind the need to protect the child with the disability. Jealousy and anger are common feelings. Parents can help a school-age child adjust and accept the sibling by encouraging honest communication about feelings. Parents may give their children a journal or a diary so they have a special place to express their thoughts and feelings. Letting children share their feelings about issues will occur at various stages.

Parents can initiate conversations by asking questions such as, "Tell me a thought or feeling you had today," or "I am wondering what you are thinking about." This type of open interest can elicit conversation and listening. Listening with an empathic ear helps validate and support feelings and thoughts. To be a good listener, set time aside, make good eye contact with the child, try not to interrupt, acknowledge feelings and give advice sparingly. If the child says, "I hate Emily's wheelchair," parents can respond by saying, "I know that you feel embarrassed by the way it looks, but it helps Emily get to the places she wants to go to." This statement validates the child's feeling of embarrassment and provides an explanation, instead of making light of the child's feeling and causing him to suppress his true thoughts. Emotions do not hurt if they are brought out in the open. They can hurt if they are suppressed, cut off or stuffed inside. Parents don't want their children to hurt and so may want to fix their pain or take it away. When parents say, "Oh, it's not so bad, stop whining," or "You shouldn't feel angry," the next time the child has a feeling, he may want to try to please the parents by not sharing the thought because it was discounted previously. There will be times when children will say things that will seem unacceptable to parents. When feelings become overwhelming, it helps to take a deep breath and step away from the situation before exploding with an inappropriate response. It is okay to offer a nonjudgmental statement such as, "I just don't know what to say, except it sounds like you are hurting and this is really hard for you." This lets the child know that she is supported. Feelings are not something with which you agree or disagree. Observing the feeling and reporting it back to the child helps the child know that you are focusing your attention and relating to what he is sharing. Parents can express their feelings and thoughts to their children as well. A statement such as, "I'm scared about John's surgery too, but I know we will get through it" expresses the parent's feelings with positive reassurance. By sharing feelings, parents are validating that expressing thoughts is okay. This helps children know that everyone has feelings and it is good to share them.

Parents can offer age-appropriate explanations about the disability. Here is one example: "Samantha has cerebral palsy. When she was born, part of her brain did not get enough oxygen or air. The part which didn't get enough air is the part that controls her walking and talking. This is why she has trouble walking and talking. She has to wear a brace on her leg to help her walk. She goes to physical and speech therapy to help her walk and talk. Cerebral palsy is not contagious. You can't catch it."

Explanations in terms they can understand will enable the children to understand what cerebral palsy is and what the treatment plan and goals are. They get reassurance that it is not contagious and they did not cause the disability.

Parents can offer periodic reassurance to help their other children know what is going on. If the sibling has to be taken for medical tests or assessments, it is important to let the other children know where the family is going for the tests as well as the reasons and when they will return. This helps to lessen the siblings' fear of the unknown.

Parents can help decrease jealousy by spending time with each child. The family can encourage siblings to pursue their outside interests and hobbies. They can also encourage their children to invite people over to play and spend the night. The family can bring the child with the special needs, when possible, on errands and family outings to help siblings come to a level of acceptance.

The Siblings

Teenagers face complex changes. They mature intellectually, form their own opinions and begin to think in abstract terms. Their feelings change rapidly from moment to moment. They are going through physical changes and experience a range of feelings regarding their sexuality. They are developing a sense of self separate from parental values. They often experience a conflict between the need to belong to a group and the need to be seen as a unique individual. They worry about what their friends will think and say. Teens are often concerned with how they look and the opinions of their peer group. All teens are embarrassed by their families at some point. This is no exception in a family with special needs.

Listening to teens with empathy helps to validate and support their concerns. The family can encourage all members to air their grievances, confront unfair feelings and solve conflicts. Family meetings can be helpful ways to enable all members to discuss issues and find ways to solve problems. All teens need time to pursue their own interests and activities, as well as to spend time with their friends. They also need to have time with their families.

Young adults worry about passing on a genetic link to their offspring. They worry that their children may have a disability. They have concerns regarding future plans with the child with the disability. They worry who will take care of this child after their parents die. Parents can ease some of their worries by having an open discussion relating as much as they know at present about future plans for the child with special needs. They can provide specific information regarding genetic inheritance.

All children experience sibling rivalry as a normal part of growing up. In special needs families there is a tendency for parents to want to protect the child with the disability from this. The normal fighting which occurs in all families may be discouraged. Parents can offer to mediate a dispute while encouraging the children to work out as many differences on their own as possible. Allowing the children to solve their own problems encourages independence.

The family may face discrimination when people begin to ask questions about the disability. Others may say things out of ignorance which will seem cruel. This causes embarrassment for siblings of all ages. Parents can become role models by using an embarrassing or uncomfortable moment as an example to teach their children how to deal with comments from strangers.

Dr. Jean Lerner, a psychotherapist suggests that families with special needs become "family-centered" rather than "child-centered." When the focus is placed on all family members, self-esteem grows. The siblings are given as much time and attention as the child who has the special need. Everyone is given equal amounts of responsibility at home. All are encouraged to pursue their own interests and activities to meet individual needs in and out of the family. If the child with the disability becomes the center of the family, others' needs go neglected. It is important to allow all the children in the family to take care of as much as they can independently. Taking over tasks that children can do for themselves interferes with the child's ability to reach his full potential. Mutual interdependence encourages family members to ask for help when necessary while enabling self-help skills.

Siblings can be involved in the care of the brother or sister with the disability but they cannot become a substitute parent. They can be taught to love and care about others without depriving them of their own lives, friends and social outings.

Support groups throughout the country have been started to provide support to siblings. One is the Sibling Information Network. It provides a bibliography of children's literature and journal articles for siblings of children with disabilities, lists of support services, as well as information about starting a sibling support group.

Tony is seven years old and has cerebral palsy. His brother, Bobby, who has Williams Syndrome and is mentally retarded, hits Tony and talks "mean" to him. Tony often feels embarrassed by some of the "weird" things Bobby does.

Becca's daughter, Shana, was born with congenital anomalies of her arm and leg. She is mobility-impaired. She can't climb stairs, pump on a bike or walk long distances. Shana's brother, Joel, has autism. According to their mother, raising two children with disabilities brought its challenges and rewards. Becca feels that Shana is one of the siblings who felt she gained from the experience of having a brother with a severe disability, rather than having been

The Siblings

hurt by the experience. She has defended him and explained his autism since she was four years old. She is compassionate and self-motivated. There were times when Shana was embarrassed by Joel's behavior. The family talked openly about their feelings. If Joel were going to attend a family outing and Shana did not want to go because she feared Joel would make strange noises and embarrass her, they discussed her feelings and chose options.

Sara is a six-year-old girl who has epilepsy. She has an older sister who is ten. Sara's mother treats both children equally, encouraging their independence. When the family wants to motivate Sara to try new things, they involve everyone at home as well as friends. They hold family meetings to discuss issues such as setting limits, disciplining and adapting rules.

Suggestions

- Communicate feelings and actively listen to concerns. Set aside time, make eye contact, do not interrupt, do acknowledge feelings, give advice sparingly.
- Explain the disability to siblings in terms which are age-appropriate. This conversation will continue over time as the needs of the child with the disability change. Issues will change as brothers and sisters mature.
- Focus on a family-centered home where the attention is placed on all members, rather than a child-centered home.
- Spend time with each child in the family. Play a game, take a walk, talk together, read a book, do chores.
- Encourage all family members to pursue their own interests and activities.

Chapter Five

THE GRANDPARENTS/EXTENDED FAMILY

Grandparents grieve for their adult child as well as for the child with the disability. They experience the stages of grief: shock, denial, bargaining, anger, guilt and acceptance, just as the parents. They may blame their adult children, themselves and the physicians. They may offer home remedies and advice. [19]

Grandparents may be removed from the situation because they live far away. They may remove themselves if they are not ready to deal with it. In most cases, grandparents and the extended family are not involved with daily care of the child and come to terms with the situation at a slower pace. This may cause stress for the adult children, who already feel isolated and strained from the overwhelming responsibilities. Some extended family members may become part of the problem.[20] They may say hurtful things about the child with the disability and stay away. Some relatives may find the situation too difficult to understand and accept.

Byron is an eleven-year-old boy who has autism. His family has had to face its share of misconceptions and prejudice within the community as well as with the extended family. Some family members have been accepting of Byron but others have not. Some have misinterpreted his behavior as "undisciplined, sick, spoiled and crazy." His mother feels that her son has to face more prejudice because he has no obvious physical disability, which seems to be accepted more readily than hidden disabilities, such as autism.

When the extended family provides support it makes a difference and helps the family gain strength.

The Grandparents/Extended Family

Bettina is a ten-year-old girl who has cerebral palsy, is mentally retarded and has seizures. Her mother feels that they have a very close extended family who provides lots of support. They treat Bettina like a "normal" child. Bettina has four aunts, eight uncles, lots of cousins and grandparents who she sees often. Sometimes, her aunt and grandparents ask her mother about her seizures and if she will ever get over them.

Parents can help extended family members accept the child with the disability by giving them time to grieve. Parents can provide information to help them understand the nature of the disability as well as the treatment plan and goals. Knowledge alleviates some of the fear about the unknown. Information can be updated as the child's situation changes. The parents may provide information about the grieving process to the extended family so they understand what they are feeling. They can be encouraged to discuss their feelings with their adult children, friends, clergy, counselors or in a support group. There are many parent support groups which provide services for extended family members.

It is helpful to remember that extended family members will not feel the same feelings at the same time as the parents of the child with disability. Acceptance of the difference of opinions and feelings may lessen expectations on the part of the adult children.

There are many ways extended family members can provide support. Grandparents can offer to listen with an empathic attitude without giving advice. When people ask what they can do to help, they often do not know what the family needs, but they want to be supportive. The family is often exhausted and has difficulty meeting basic needs. Relatives can offer to cook meals, pick up groceries or medicine, take the other children in the family on outings, or accompany the mother or father to a therapy session for moral support.

For relatives who live far away, it is even more difficult for them to understand the nature of the family situation. They do not see the children on a daily basis so their level of acceptance may take much longer. The parents can keep them updated by providing information, writing letters about the progress of the children, as well as by sending pictures. This helps to keep the lines of communication open.

A Grandparents' Story

The grandparents of a three-year-old girl with cerebral palsy describe their family relationship and struggles to adjust. Their grandchild is a "sweet, lovable, pretty child with a great disposition." At home, she loves to watch Barney. She loves to have books read to her and to look at the pictures. She likes to have tea parties with her play dishes.

Their grandchild has moderate cerebral palsy. She is unable to walk, is weak in her trunk and has limited use of her left arm and hand. She is just beginning to talk. She attends a private nursery school where none of the other children in her classroom are handicapped. She is learning to imitate the other children. Her teachers are a great source of encouragement.

The parents and grandparents have been open with all their friends about discussing disabilities. The child's family encourages her independence by using lots of praise. Limits and discipline are set as if their grandchild has no disability. However, they explain, there is very little need for setting limits, because she cannot crawl very well. The parents measure her progress in small increments. Balancing independence without attempts to rescue is left up to her parents. The grandparents balance as best as they can.

The relationship between their two-year-old grandchild and her three-year-old sibling is normal: loving and jealous.

The most difficult thing for the grandparents is being around children of their granddaughter's age who are not handicapped. It is also difficult for them to accept the fact that the cerebral palsy will become less of a handicap but will not go away completely. They also tend to become impatient with the girl's progress. Additionally, the grandparents feel that people tend to view those with physical disabilities or chronic illnesses as not being normal.

They offer suggestions to other grandparents, telling them to maintain a sense of hope regarding the future of their grandchild. No one can look into the future and tell you what your grandchild will be capable of in ten years. Take care of your other grandchildren. Do not neglect them. Stay informed by reading available books and magazines on the subject. Find support for yourself by talking with doctors, therapists, teachers and other grandparents who have a child who has a disability. Take your grandchild around other children. Children seem to be the happiest when they are with other children. Try not to compare your grandchild with other children with disabilities. Each child is unique. Medical science has made great strides in recent years in regard to medications, surgery and therapy.

Time is on your side. Support your adult child. Offer to take their children on outings, to appointments; invite them to dinner. You need each other for emotional support. Try to lead as normal a life as possible. Discuss your grandchild's disability openly with relatives and friends, especially if they ask. You will find that the more informed they are, the better able they are to deal with you and your grandchild. Your feelings of sadness and desperation are normal. Talk about your feelings with your spouse and close friends. Do not blame yourself because your grandchild has special needs. Because of your grandchild's disability, you will meet a lot of nice people whom you would not have met otherwise. Enjoy their friendship.

A Grandmother's Grief

"Our granddaughter has cerebral palsy. How do [we] deal with this, the dreaded nightmare, that something is wrong with our grandchild? Why didn't she sit up without support when she was six months old? I did not want to worry my daughter and ask her. I just thought she was a little slow in her physical development. Maybe the doctor and my daughter were wrong in calculating her due date. Each time we saw her, it became more noticeable that she just wasn't doing things as her sisters had done at her age. My husband and I discussed it and we kept saying she'll be fine. We watched the children when she was one. She was crawling and sitting on her knees. When I gave her a bath, I had to support her back as you would an infant. I had to strap her in her high chair because she still could not sit without help. She pulled herself up to try and walk, but could only walk holding on. I then noticed that her right foot was not flat on the floor but always on her toe. But I still did not say anything to my daughter, and kept telling myself she was just a little behind schedule. At the age of fourteen months, she still was not making any progress sitting or walking. I finally called my daughter and told her about our concerns. Then she told me that she and her husband had been worried about her and had repeatedly told the pediatrician about the problem. The pediatrician's answer was, "She'll get there." My daughter took her to an orthopedic surgeon, who looked at her and immediately said it was not an orthopedic problem but a neurological problem. That's when it started: the fear, the tears, the unacceptable, that something was terribly wrong with our grandbaby. Who do I cry for first, my beautiful grandbaby or my beautiful daughter?

"You want to say this is not true, but deep in your heart you've known there was something wrong for months. Where do we go from here? The luxury of tears has to stop. We must go on with the daily job of living. How do we do this with our hearts so full of sorrow? My adult child needs my support. She has to think that I'm strong so she too will be strong.

"Grandma and Grandpa will be the best support system that we can be. We will always be there when needed. We will try very hard not to be interfering. We will take our other grandkids when we can.

"We have known that diagnosis of cerebral palsy for seven months now. I have accepted the fact that our grandchild has a disability. I don't know if Grandpa has. I have stopped trying to answer the question "why?" or questioning whether the doctors were at fault or asking was the hospital at fault. We probably will never know. But what we do know is that we have been blessed with a wonderful little girl."

Suggestions

- Grandparents grieve for their adult children as well as their grandchildren. To help extended family members deal with grieving, the adult children can give them information about the stages of grief.
- Encourage grandparents and other extended family members to talk about their feelings with a friend, clergy, counselor,

The Grandparents/Extended Family

support group or with their adult children. Provide the name of a local family support group to the extended family members.
- Give extended family members literature about the disability so they can understand the nature of the condition as well as the treatment plans and goals.
- Grandparents, friends and other relatives can support the family by helping them take care of basic needs. Some suggested ways to help include: cooking a meal, running an errand, picking up groceries or medical supplies, taking the other children in the family on an outing or going to a medical appointment with the child.
- Extended family can offer support by listening with empathy.

Chapter Six

FOSTERING INDEPENDENCE FOR CHILDREN WITH DISABILITIES

Promoting safe independence, when possible, is a balancing act. Knowing when to give children their wings is even more difficult when the child has a mental or physical disability or both. Children with severe disabilities must rely heavily upon others. The reality of such dependence should not be minimized. For some children, it may be nearly impossible to maintain a sense of independence. When possible, developing goals which support individuals to lead their lives as independently as possible helps to foster self-sufficiency.

Developing goals to enhance independence varies according to each child and family. Independence does not necessarily mean that a person must do all things alone. Interdependence is a more appropriate relationship: people depending on one another for support and assistance. Interdependence focuses on mutually empathic relationships where each person cares about the well-being of the other. Family members are encouraged to express their thoughts, feelings and concerns and take responsibility to become as self-reliant as possible.

Jane is a thirty-four-year-old woman who is a physical therapist and has cerebral palsy. Her parents allowed her to do anything within reason. They never told her "no" or "that's too tiring." Her parents thought she was a "superior" child and they made Jane believe it. Her parents reinforced how special and valued she was. Caldwell, a thirty-eight-year-old teacher, was born with missing fingers, one foot and missing toes on the other due to thalidomide

Fostering Independence for Children with Disabilities

syndrome. She described her family as "one full of life, acceptance, encouragement and a positive attitude." They were the most positive force in her life and the reason she is the person she is today. Caldwell's parents allowed her to try. They were never shocked or amazed when she accomplished something. They were always encouraging. They treated her like any other family member. Caldwell thought they treated her with a little more tolerance than they probably should have, as she was "spoiled and sheltered."

Brent is a thirty-three-year-old deaf man who is a language support specialist with deaf students. He had supportive parents who believed in him and knew that he had the ability to communicate with other people. His parents gave him the love, support, praise and encouragement he needed to cope and succeed.

The formation of the self-concept begins with relationships with family and is influenced as one gets older by friends, peers, teachers and others. How a person is viewed by significant others contributes to a person's feelings about himself. For children with special needs, self-concept is influenced by relationships as well as the age of onset and the severity of the disability, cognitive skills, emotional or physical abilities, the amount of dependence upon others and the degree to which independence is possible.

To develop healthy self-esteem, a child needs to feel a sense of personal independence, personal responsibility and a realistic definition of self, while being given equal opportunities for growth in a positive environment. Nothing deflates self-esteem faster than being limited by an overprotective parent, being denied training because of sex or disability or being looked down upon by others.

There is some evidence that boys and girls who have disabilities may be raised a little differently.[22] Some research indicates that the parents of girls were less likely to encourage and expect self-sufficiency and community living than the parents of boys.[23] If expectations are reduced, this may inadvertently lead to lower self-esteem, dependence, unemployment and poverty for the child as he or she becomes an adult. Boys and girls should be given every equal opportunity to become as independent as possible. It is important to raise boys and girls with the same expectations and provide equal opportunities for growth. Women with disabilities face prejudice because of gender and special needs.[24] Women with special needs are viewed in stereotypical terms by close friends, family and other significant people who are involved in their lives. People sometimes see women as being more dependent. They are not given credit for being able to participate in community life, having a job, intimacy and sexual relationships or becoming a parent. Parents can help their female children reach their full potential by being cautious of their own attitudes and images. Getting to know adult women with disabilities can help provide role models for the family.

Parents who produce children with high self-esteem show love and acceptance on a daily basis, with affection and concern without criticism. They set clear rules which are enforced in a democratic, fair manner.[25] There are some suggested guidelines for enhancing positive self-esteem and producing people who are as self-sufficient as possible.[26] Parents in these families set realistic expectations for their children. They listen with empathy and allow for the expression of honest and open communication. Children are encouraged to pursue their own activities and interests and social skills. They help motivate their children to try new skills and take risks. Parents offer realistic praise and set attainable goals. They introduce their children to role models. They respect everyone's right to privacy. They provide opportunities so everyone in the family can reach their full potential and participate in community life when possible.

Expectations which emphasize positive abilities to achieve allow children to learn independence and competence. It is important to acknowledge the child's realistic limitations but push for the best. Allowing children to do things their own way is important as it enables them to think about their options and come up with solutions. Encouraging children to try is important.

Samantha is three and has cerebral palsy. She has trouble dressing and undressing because of her mobility problem. There are certain things she is expected to do in this task. She can choose her own clothes. They are in low drawers which she can reach. She can pull her shirt over her head and put her arms through. She can't stand to pull up her pants, but she can pull the pants over her legs. This task is broken down into small steps, which allows Samantha to do what she can. This helps to increase her sense of

Fostering Independence for Children with Disabilities

self-reliance. For older children, parents can define the task and steps to reach the goal, ensuring that the child takes as much responsibility as possible to complete the task.

Allowing the child to become a contributing member of the family, with assigned chores and household duties, helps to make the child feel self-sufficient. When the child can be responsible for his own care, let him. Tasks such as dressing, feeding, brushing teeth and combing hair help a child know that he is self-reliant. It is important to allow each child to complete tasks without constant help, reminders and suggestions, even if a parent could complete the task faster and more efficiently.

Bettina is a ten-year-old girl who has cerebral palsy and is mentally retarded. Her mother tries to promote Bettina's independence without attempts to rescue but finds it very difficult. It took a long time, but she realizes that if she did everything for Tina, the child would never try. Now, she gives Tina lots of praise for doing something successfully on her own. Eleven-year-old Byron has autism and his parents feel they need to rescue him in social situations. They step in if Byron misinterprets the actions of others. If children are playing a game of tag and they try to involve Byron, he may think a tag is a push or an assault. His parents try to explain the action to him so that he understands what to do if it happens again. His parents calmly talk about the misunderstanding. When Byron tries a new activity, his parents coach the situation first. They review the scenario so Byron will be prepared and know what to expect. They teach him ways to handle difficult situations. They set goals for him by trying to focus on the attainable. They use behavior modification and give rewards for following rules at home. They take allowance and Nintendo time away for not following rules.

Providing opportunities which enable children to learn new tasks encourages risk-taking. They learn that it is okay to make mistakes and fail. Teaching skills which allow for decision-making and choices help children become better equipped to determine their way in the community as they grow. Opportunities which provide small age-appropriate choices, such as what to wear and what to eat, progress to choosing people with whom they wish to associate as well as in which activities they want to participate.

As children grow, it is important to allow them to choose their friends, activities and learn to struggle with new situations they may encounter. Parents can teach their children how to handle struggles, which empowers them to make decisions on their own. Helping children find meaning in difficult situations enables them to learn how to handle the next situation.

Jane is a thirty-four-year-old woman who has cerebral palsy. When she was a little girl, she wanted to go on a five-mile bike ride with her friends. She had never ridden that far. Her parents were worried and afraid that she might tire out. They encouraged her to try it, telling her that if she got tired at any point, she could call and they would pick her up. Eleven-year-old Siobhan has severe mental retardation but her parents let her do as much as possible. Motivating her to try new things hasn't been a problem because she likes to try. To encourage her independence, Siobhan has started going away on weekend outings with other children. These trips are arranged by the community health board. It has been difficult for her mother to let her go, because she feels no one else is able to take care of Siobhan's needs like she can. Her mother, however, knows that it is essential to let her daughter live as normal a life as possible.

Empathy, honesty and open communication in the family promote healthy feelings about one's self-esteem. There is a balance between not making the child's disability the center of attention while discussing it honestly.[27] Parents can emphasize the child's personality and strengths while reminding them that they have things in common with other children as well.

Helping children understand how the disability affects them is important. Parents can describe the disability using medical and familiar terminology. The information should be honest as well as age- and developmentally-appropriate. All children will not be able to understand the implications of a special need due to their developmental age and the severity of the disability. Issues will change as the child grows. Parents can listen to their child's concerns using empathy. Children's concerns will be different than those of their parents.[28] Children experience their own stages of grieving apart from parents' feelings. A parent can assure the child that the disability is not contagious, nor anyone's fault and that

Fostering Independence for Children with Disabilities

sometimes things happen for no understandable reason. They may experience wanting to be like other children by refusing to wear hearing aids, use crutches, braces, wheelchairs, etc. They may become angry due to the attention which they receive because of their disability.

Actively listen to a child's concerns without giving advice, no matter how difficult it may be to hear. Help the child make sense of another's stares or comments. Reassure the child that sometimes people stare because they do not understand or have not had exposure to people with special needs. Provide explanations which are honest in terms that the child will understand.

Shana is a college student who was born missing parts of her fingers and toes. When Shana was little, she asked her mother why the doctor removed her fingers. She didn't think of herself as disabled. When she started preschool, children were cruel to her. They called her names and wouldn't hold her hand. Her parents felt that it was important to empower Shana to define herself. Her parents told her that her hands and feet belonged to her and she did not have to talk about them to anyone if she didn't want to. But Shana was encouraged to talk about her feelings regarding her disability.

Danielle's mother described her disability to her by using the word delayed. Danielle does not talk about her disability to other children. If others comment or stare at her, her mother redirects Danielle. Sara's mother has told her that she has epilepsy, which causes her to have seizures. Sara does not see herself like other children who have epilepsy. Tony's mother began to explain his cerebral palsy once he started asking questions. She explained how the CP happened and how it affects everyone in different ways. Tony tells his friends he can't walk because he was born too early and his muscles were damaged. Matthew's mother explained his hearing impairment by telling him that he wears hearing aids to hear just as others wear glasses so they can see. If a stranger questions Matthew about his hearing aids, he tells them that he wears them to help him hear better. Bettina's mother described her cerebral palsy and mental retardation by telling her that she may not be able to walk or talk like others now, but someday she will. She has also told Bettina that she will need help for quite awhile.

AFTER YOUR CHILD'S DIAGNOSIS

At some point, children are made aware of their differences. They may come home from school one day and begin to ask their parents why they are different. The child may express his concerns at this point. Children feel and respond in their own way and in their own time-frame. They will have both positive and negative feelings about their special needs.

Tony, who is six, has cerebral palsy and his parents told him about his disability when he began to ask questions. His mother told him that when he was nine months old, he was diagnosed with cerebral palsy due to damage to his central nervous system. They told him that CP affects everyone differently. Tony's CP affects his leg muscles. Tony has physical therapy, which he does not like. He has shared his feelings about it with his mother. He doesn't like to be stretched because it hurts. At times, he feels angry when he has to go. At night, he wears splints to help position his legs. He doesn't like to wear them, but he knows they help, so he does. There are times when he gets frustrated with other children who stare or make comments about his disability. He has times when he feels proud of himself. Tony loves to play football with the help of his walker. He considers himself a pretty good football player, baseball player and swimmer. He is proud of his reading and math skills.

When children do express themselves, it is important to validate their feelings and provide support. Parents often want to fix the sad feeling by saying, "Cheer up, it's not that bad." This comment ignores the feeling. By acknowledge the feeling, "I know it makes you feel sad that you can't run like your friends," parents are providing support.

Getting children involved in support groups can be helpful. They can meet other children who have disabilities. They can share ideas, feelings, and gain strength and support by being with other children who share a common bond. Family support groups often provide social outings for the entire family as well as support groups for the children.

Activities, interests and social skills are very important in developing a sense of identity. Parents need to ensure that a child has many opportunities to develop his or her social skills in a variety of settings. Allowing a child to find an activity that he or she

Fostering Independence for Children with Disabilities

enjoys accentuates his or her talents, which promotes confidence and positive self-esteem.

There are many activities that are sponsored by local organizations which have programs for children with special needs. Children with disabilities may participate in regular programs or specific programs designed for people who have special needs. (See Leisure Section of Resource Guide). One example is Winners on Wheels, which provides activities for children between the ages of seven and fourteen. WOW believes in helping children take risks and solve problems in a safe learning environment while building self-esteem. It provides opportunities to participate in wheelchair sports, meet adults with disabilities and share common concerns. The North American Riders For The Handicapped Association is another organization; it has 525 riding centers across the United States offering therapeutic horseback riding for people who have disabilities. NARHA will send parents a list of centers in their state, including address, phone number and contact person. Boy and Girl Scouts offer a variety of programs for children with disabilities. The National Handicapped Sports and Recreation Association, the National Wheelchair Athletic Association, the United Cerebral Palsy Athletic Association and The Special Olympics are just some of the organizations which provide information about recreation for people with disabilities. There are a variety of camps which also offer opportunities for recreation.

Giving children ample opportunities to participate in community life provides a sense of personal growth, a sense of belonging and a feeling of inclusion. Six-year-old Sara has epilepsy but her mother encourages her to participate in the activities she enjoys. Sara swims, plays with neighbors and loves ballet. The family rides bikes together. They play board games, cards and entertain friends and family. Danielle is an eight-year-old girl who has cerebral palsy and is developmentally delayed. Her family spends their spare time camping, skating, going to movies and bike-riding. Jonathan is a nine-year-old boy who has cerebral palsy. He loves reading and writing. When he was eight, his family helped him publish two short stories and a poem.

Motivation, praise and goal-setting reinforce positive behavior. Giving praise for persisting when things are difficult or slow helps a child feel motivated to keep trying. Sara's parents set goals in steps, one at a time. Allowing a child to enjoy his or her successes slowly rather than hurrying on to the next goal or task allows the child to appreciate it without feeling pressure to overexcel or superachieve.

Fair and consistent discipline, which sets clear limits and rules, promotes positive decision-making and understanding that there are consequences for good and bad choices. Teaching limits with consistency is important. Rules with reasons help to teach lessons: "Don't hit the cat because you will hurt her." Provide choices or alternatives such as "You can't draw on the wall because it won't come off. Here are some crayons and paper instead." Distraction and ignoring poor behavior helps stop it without arguing. If a child has a tantrum, he can be removed from the room or ignored until it stops. Catch children being good and tell them about it. There should be logical consequences for behavior which is unacceptable. Aaron is nine and has autism. His parents treat him like any normal child. They demand a lot out of him and they encourage him with praise, guidance and love. They set strict limits and discipline by sticking with a routine.

To encourage positive self-esteem, it is important to not overindulge, spoil or pity. Those qualities only serve to create people who do not feel confident in their abilities. Sara's mother knows that other people are afraid to correct her daughter or discipline her when she needs it because they are afraid that Sara might have a seizure. Sara's mother knows this won't happen. It is important to not to use the disability as an excuse for not disciplining.

Role models serve to enable people to share common experiences, inspiration, hope and encouragement. To have a role model to look up to during times of doubt or insecurity provides a source of encouragement and empathy. Association with people who share a common bond helps to decrease the sense of isolation and the feelings of being different. Many organizations and support groups provide opportunities for families to meet adults with disabilities. United Cerebral Palsy has a mentoring project which links children up with adults who have cerebral palsy. The National Council of Independent Living Programs has information about local centers which provide peer counseling and mentoring to people

Fostering Independence for Children with Disabilities

who have disabilities, as well as independent living skills, advocacy and education. The Networking Project for Women and Girls with Disabilities provides information to individuals and groups about starting a mentoring program in their communities. The Handicapped Organization for Women is another resource which helps empower women through education and advocacy. (The Resource Guide lists addresses.)

The right to privacy is often taken away from individuals with disabilities. If their disability is apparent or visible, they are stared at, comments are made and questions are sometimes asked. Each person has the right to privacy and confidentiality. Who and what people with disabilities choose to explain is a personal decision based upon the nature of the relationship. Matthew is an eight-year-old boy who is hearing impaired. When he is at school, children often question him about his hearing aids, which embarrasses him. Tony has cerebral palsy. Some children at school have asked him questions about his inability to walk. They have said mean things and have hurt Tony's feelings. There are times when he doesn't want to talk about his disability. He has friends who have disabilities and this helps him feel accepted for who he is. They don't ask questions about his cerebral palsy. At home children have the right to privacy as well. They should be able to have quiet time when they need it. Knocking on doors when they are closed gives a message of respect.

Community concerns and future planning for children with disabilities requires active advocacy and participation of the parents. The family must ensure that the child's needs are being met so that he or she will have every opportunity to become as self-sufficient as possible. The family must work with schools and other agencies to ensure that the child's future needs are being met. Transition training for teens should include exploring options for future employment, coordination with adult service providers, postsecondary education and participation in community activities. The options for living arrangements must be explored. Financial planning for the child's future must be taken into account. Wills, trusts and Social Security benefits, which will provide for the child's care, must be safeguarded, and his or her eligibility requirements met. (See Chapters Eight and Eleven for specific information.)

Sexuality should be discussed with children who are able to understand. Sexuality is an integral part of one's self-concept. Teaching children about caring, loving and intimacy lays the groundwork for a positive sexual identity. Children with disabilities are no exception. People with mild to severe disabilities are capable of having physical intimacy. There are myths and stereotypes about people with disabilities which negate their sexual desire and needs.[29] It is still sometimes assumed that people with disabilities do not have a sexual identity. It is important to give children with disabilities information about safe sex, birth control, love and intimacy. Parents need to have an open mind when questions are being asked. They can use factual information with accurate body terms. They can bring up sexual issues in family conversations rather than scheduling a talk. Parents can discuss what appropriate touching is to ensure that their children understand that their bodies belong to them. Parents should warn children about the dangers of inappropriate touch which comes with sexual abuse and molestation. Teaching children to say no and to tell a safe adult if anyone touches them sexually or if anyone asks them to do something that feels strange should be discussed. Parents can request sexual education materials from the Planned Parenthood Federation, the Sex Information and Education Council of the United States and the Coalition on Sexuality and Disability.

Suggestions

- To increase self-esteem, provide children with a sense of personal independence, personal responsibility and a realistic definition of self.
- Give children information about their disability which is age- and developmentally-appropriate. Use medical terms as well as the words your child uses.
- Raise boys and girls with the same expectations and provide equal opportunities for growth. Contact an organization for mentoring program.

Fostering Independence for Children with Disabilities

- Contact organizations to locate recreation and leisure activities.
- Provide information about sexuality. Contact an organization to obtain sex education information.

Chapter Seven

ISSUES FOR ADOLESCENTS WITH DISABILITIES

Teenage years are turbulent, critical years. Physical and emotional changes are overwhelming. Teens naturally pull away from family and move toward their peers and socialization. An unsteady self-esteem and confusing feelings contribute to the uncertainties. Teens with disabilities face additional pressures. Their attitudes about their special needs are related to the severity and age of onset of the disability, cognitive skills, emotional or physical abilities, the degree of dependence and autonomy and their level of acceptance of their differences. They often experience the same need to belong to a peer group and feel confident about their ability to do so, but find that this may not be possible because of physical limitations or intellectual disabilities.[30]

During adolescence, teens change intellectually. Some have the ability to reason and think in abstract terms. Their opinions and understanding about their world changes. They struggle to find a balance between the need to belong to their peer group and maintain a sense of uniqueness. For a teenager with a disability, this process becomes even more complicated. Some compare their own abilities to those of friends who do not have physical or intellectual limitations. If they have not come to terms with their disability and reached some point of acceptance of their own limitations, it makes it painful to watch friends participate in the things they cannot. Driving, walking, running, reaching for things, carrying, and participating in sports and activities are some of the everyday things that teens with disabilities wish they could do.[31] When they see others do these things with ease it causes some teens with special needs to feel sad and frustrated.

Issues for Adolescents with Disabilities

Friendship is an important part of the teenage years. Having a good friend with whom you can share secret thoughts and feelings is part of being a teenager. Some friends may not know how to behave with a person who has a disability because they haven't had much experience with people who have special needs. They may try to help too much because they do not know how many things their friend is really capable of doing himself. They may offer pity instead of respect because they feel sorry for their friend who cannot participate in many activities. Friends may not be honest about their true feelings if a disagreement occurs. They may worry about hurting their friend's feelings more than they should. They may see the person with the disability as being frail or unable to handle normal criticism. Instead of sharing their true feelings and thoughts, they think they are protecting their friend if they remain silent. Protecting a person with a disability perpetuates their feelings of helplessness and decreases their sense of esteem. When possible, it is up to the person with the disability to let their friends know what they need help with and what things they can do on their own. It is also up to them to let their friends know they can take honesty, even if it may hurt their feelings. They have to reassure their friends that they are not frail and they won't break. If this is known up-front, it helps to alleviate some of the uncomfortable feelings for everyone involved. The person with the disability can tell their friends that he does not want pity and he will let them know when he needs help. He can let them know that he appreciates their concern.

Sometimes a person's disability can cause isolation. The isolation may occur due to the severity of the disability and the inability to participate with other people on a regular basis. It may also occur because of negative attitudes of people regarding disabilities. Isolation can lead to poor social skills, which perpetuates uncomfortable feelings in social situations. When possible, it is important to provide teens with as many opportunities to socialize as they can to prevent isolation from occurring. Getting involved with organizations which provide support for people with disabilities is one way to minimize isolation. There are many teen organizations which provide activities. Getting involved in a sport is a good way to stay fit, be with other people and increase self-esteem.

The National Wheelchair Athletic Association, The Special Olympics and The National Handicapped Sports and Recreation Association are examples of places to receive information and referral for participation in sports. The family can involve the teen's physical or occupational therapist in suggesting ways athletic equipment can be made to fit the needs of the person. They can also suggest ways to enhance the sports activity to meet the needs of therapy. The National Center for Youth with Disabilities provides a list of services for teenagers as well as support groups and a newsletter. Global Teen Club International is an organization of ethnically diverse and socially aware teens which publishes newsletters, articles and stories written by Global Teen members.

Family relationships change during the teenage years. Teens often feel as if they are on an emotional roller coaster. Their moods can swing from anger to sadness to insecurity to embarrassment in one minute. Some teenagers try to balance the pressures to conform and belong to their peer group while trying to figure out their self-image apart from their parents' values. They want their independence from their family, yet continue to need reassurance that they are an integral part of the family.

Teens with disabilities face additional feelings which result from their perceptions of how they are treated by others. Guilt, resentment and helplessness are common feelings.[32] Some teens express feelings of guilt because they feel that they would like to be able to help more around the house but they are limited in what they can do. They may feel like a burden because their family spends time helping them with tasks that require assistance. The may feel guilty because of the expenses connected with medical care due to the disability. They may also feel guilty for not living up to parental expectations or accomplishing what they think they should accomplish. Parents can help their teens by having realistic expectations and reassuring them that their feelings are normal. If the teenager wants to talk about his feelings related to guilt, the parent may respond by saying, "I know it must be very difficult for you to want to do more at home and you feel guilty because of it, but maybe there are some things you can do." This helps to validate the feeling of guilt but also provides a plan to help increase the child's self-esteem. Parents can help their teenager

Issues for Adolescents with Disabilities

focus on the things he or she can do rather than looking at the things he or she cannot. They can make a list of household responsibilities for each child in the family so everyone feels they are contributing to the family in equal ways. The roles of the family members should be updated as they grow. Teenagers need to feel that they have a mature status within the family. They want to make decisions and have others respect their opinions and follow through with their ideas. To encourage participation in family activities, each child should be seen as a unique individual who is respected for his talent and ideas. Having teens contribute to organizing a family event, such as cooking a meal or preparing parts of a meal, planning a menu, planning a family outing such as choosing the movie or making a dinner reservation, helps validate that they are important. This increases a sense of belonging and boosts self-confidence.

When others in the family take over for the person with the special needs, it is resented and then can lead to feelings of helplessness. Teens with disabilities want the chance to be as independent as possible. Sometimes it takes a little longer to get something accomplished if the person has mobility problems. Others may think that it is easier to do it themselves rather than waiting for the person with the disability to do it. When this happens, the person who continually takes over ends up resenting him for the extra work. It can become a vicious cycle. To alleviate the resentment, it is helpful to have everyone in the family discuss his feelings regarding situations which lead to resentment. It may be that the siblings resent the person with the disability because they feel they have to do more housework. They may feel that their parents focus more time and energy on their sibling because of the disability and they may resent both the parents and the sibling. The parents can validate everyone's feelings and then develop solutions which meet the family's needs. The teen with the disability can discuss ways that he can contribute to the family to feel independent. If he feels that everyone is doing too much for him, he needs to say so and come up with ways to be seen as independent.

Embarrassment is something all teens experience. They are embarrassed by their parents and their siblings. They feel that people are looking at them all of the time. For teens with special needs, feeling embarrassed is all too common.[33] This occurs because they may need more help due to mobility problems. Embarrassment may be felt by teens who have intellectual disabilities. They may need help dressing, bathing, going to the bathroom and opening doors. It may take longer to accomplish simple tasks. When they are out in public and their friends see them with their parents helping them out in the open, it leads to embarrassing feelings. Teens should be encouraged to talk about these times. Parents can listen with empathy and keep an open mind about ways this can be minimized. Together they can come up with solutions to ensure that the teen's need for privacy are respected. Teens need to feel if they close the door to their room or bathroom, that people will knock before opening it. Some teens with disabilities may need extra help with grooming. It is important that this care is received in a dignified manner which is approved by the person with the special need and his parent, attendant or nurse.

It is common for parents to become overwhelmed with their changing teenager and they won't always know how to react to their moods, friends, clothes, hairstyle or their opinions. Parents and teenagers will have different points of view. When parents show their children that they respect their decisions and appreciate them for who they are, it helps increase their child's self-esteem.

Parents should also be aware of extreme moods. Depression is a common feeling which occurs during the teenage years. Sometimes teenagers may consider suicide if they become very depressed.[34] Some signs to look for include: sleeping more, exhaustion, increased isolation, little interest in things they used to like to do, wishing they were someone else, neglect of how they look, crying for no reason, extreme weight gain or loss, feelings of helplessness or hopelessness. Parents who notice several of these signs can talk to their teen about depression and find someone with whom the teen can share his feelings. A counselor, clergy member, a support group or a friend can help with feelings of depression. When appropriate, it can be helpful to provide the teenager with a journal to express his thoughts and feelings. If journal keeping is not possible, a computer or tape recorder which is off-limits to other members of the family can become another way of recording thoughts and feelings.

Parents can discuss the dangers of smoking, drinking alcohol and taking illegal drugs. They can teach their children how to say no to their friends. Helping teens see themselves as unique individuals and finding healthy ways to belong to peer groups will help them make good decisions for themselves.

Some teens with special needs worry about their future. They worry about meeting their education needs, getting a job, having a relationship, having children and fulfilling their dreams. Parents can help their children reach the full potential by advocating for their child's needs at school and finding professional resources.

A possible resource in planning early for a child's future is looking into an independent living center. Tony Koosis is the program director at the Houston Independent Living Center. He suggests that all parents plan far in advance for their children's future after high school since there are waiting lists for federally-funded programs and services such as housing, equipment and employment training programs. Some waiting lists last up to two years. There are fewer services available and it takes longer than families realize to plan. Tony recommends that parents start researching their options when their child reaches thirteen. Parents can locate an independent living center in their area by contacting the Independent Living Center Research Utilization Program, which lists 250 independent living centers throughout the United States. This is a federally-funded program which conducts nationwide training for centers. Independent Living Centers are established by people with disabilities. They have a board made up of members who have disabilities and they provide a variety of services. They provide peer counseling to help people come to terms with their special needs and offer practical solutions. They teach self-help and adjustment skills. They provide information and referral. They will help locate resources, such as vocational training, which may include finding employment, assisting with resume and interview skills, affordable apartments and group homes, transportation services, and equipment. Independent Living Centers also provide computer access training programs and assistive technology training.

They advocate for individuals for fair treatment under the Americans with Disabilities Act.

Tony recommends that parents begin planning early through the child's Individual Education Plan (IEP). They should set clear goals and monitor that they are being met by the child's teachers. If the parents do not feel a school district is meeting their child's needs, Tony recommends locating an advocate to help. Advocacy Incorporated is an example of one federally-funded program. It is a nonprofit corporation formed to protect the legal rights of persons who are disabled and is funded through special federal legislation. It provides protection and advocacy for developmentally-disabled persons, client assistance programs for people who are receiving or seeking services funded by the Vocational Rehabilitation Act and parent training.

Teenagers Living with Special Needs

Joshua is a seventeen-year-old student in tenth grade. He is enrolled in independent study at home. He was diagnosed with nemaline myopathy, a congenital disease of the skeletal muscles, at age four.

Joshua has had to spend a good part of his growing up undergoing many surgeries on his back, hand, foot and leg. He has also been hospitalized for staph pneumonia. Joshua needs special equipment to help him with mobility as well as medical care. He wears leg braces. He uses a three-wheel scooter. He has had a tracheotomy and uses a ventilator.

He also missed a great deal of school because he was pulled out of regular classes to attend physical, occupational and speech therapy.

His family provides a great source of support and answers all of his questions regarding his special needs. He doesn't recall his parents telling him about his disability. As issues arise, he asks and they answer honestly. Joshua's brother has been and is helpful, especially when Josh needs help lifting something, getting something off a shelf and taking a bath. Joshua's family helps him feel independent. His family is realistic about the things Josh can and can't do. They allow him to try new things on his own. The most difficult thing that Joshua has tried recently is cooking.

Some things Joshua feels sad about relate to his inability to be as independent as he would like to be. He is unable to do somethings because he is ventilator dependent. This includes swimming and sleeping over at friends' homes. He finds it frustrating that he cannot do the things other boys his age do. He often feels embarrassed when his equipment falls apart. He sometimes suffers from nightmares about falling in the water and drowning. He wishes he could breathe on his own without a ventilator and be as strong as his father. He has to deal with stereotypical views from friends at school who often treat him as though he were younger than he actually is. They also think that because he has a physical disability he also has an intellectual impairment.

When Joshua is older, he would like to do something with computers in the medical field. He spends a great deal of time using his computer. He tries very hard not to let his disability get in the way of what he wants to do.

Marsha

Marsha is eighteen and attends high school. She describes herself as confident, very trustworthy, a great listener and a good advice giver. She loves to write letters, talk on the phone and watch television. She enjoys going out for dinner with her family.

Marsha's cerebral palsy affects her arms and legs. She uses a motorized wheelchair and a scooter which enables her to get around easier. She has to work extremely hard at the things she can do. Her left hand is more affected than her right. Occupational therapy has helped to strengthen her hand so that she can open and close it easily and hold things in it. Physical therapy has taught her relaxation techniques to reduce tense muscle tone, but only temporarily. She feels that physical therapy is only a temporary solution to a permanent problem.

Marsha does not remember her parents telling her about her disability. She says she was always aware of her special needs. She feels that her family has always been there for her and doesn't treat her any differently than they treat her sister. She doesn't feel that she is any different than a person without special needs. Marsha believes that because her sister treats her like a normal person she fits into any kind of situation and doesn't feel like an outcast. Marsha credits her friends and family for keeping her spirits high.

Marsha's friends are people with and without disabilities. She feels it is important to have friends with disabilities because they can relate to what she is going through. She is involved in a pen-pal program for people with special needs. She feels sometimes that her friends take advantage of her, which hurts her feelings and frustrates her when they don't keep their promises.

At first Marsha attended a special school for students with special needs. She was mainstreamed into a regular school later. She was the only disabled student in the school and the students didn't know how to approach her, so they made rude comments. But, as time went on, they accepted her for who she was.

One of the most difficult new tasks for Marsha was making the transition from an aid helping her in high school to being totally independent at home. She needs a lot of assistance. She feels at times that she has not been allowed to try new things on her own. When she goes places and finds that they are not accessible to her, she finds it very frustrating. She would like to be able to go out with her friends more often. She would like to go to more places without her parents going with her.

One of Marsha's accomplishments is performing well in school. She receives good grades and is very proud when she achieves her goals. She wants to be a social worker or counselor for young adults with special needs.

Marsha wishes someday to become fully independent with some limitations, be successful and be able to help inspire other people.

Suggestions

- Intellectual, physical and emotional changes accompany adolescent years. Acknowledging and validating feelings as well

Issues for Adolescents with Disabilities

as coming up with solutions to minimize problem areas helps to increase feelings of self-worth. When appropriate, encourage teenagers to record their feelings in a journal or on a computer or tape recorder which remains a private source of expression.

- Teach teens assertive communication to deal with family, friends and professionals. Allow them to take every opportunity to get their needs met so they can feel independent and self-reliant.
- To decrease isolation, encourage teenagers to pursue an interest in a teen group, activity or sport. Encourage them to contact an organization listed in the Resource Guide under leisure or youth activities.
- Watch for signs of depression—find a professional counselor if necessary.
- Locate an independent living center in your community early to research options for future planning.

Chapter Eight

THE SCHOOL

The quality of a child's educational experience depends on the working relationship among the school district, teachers, parents and related professionals. The goal of the team effort is to ensure that the child's educational needs are being met in the most beneficial way. It is up to the parents to make sure that the child's goals are met while monitoring his progress.

The Education for All Handicapped Children's Act of 1975 (EAHCA), also known as Public Law 94-142 or sometimes referred to as the Individuals with Disabilities Education Act (IDEA), has improved educational opportunities for children with disabilities.[35] The law does not ensure that the child will receive an "ideal educational program."[36] It only requires that the child has access to special education and services.

The law entitles students with disabilities to receive "free, appropriate education in the least restrictive environment." The education must be provided at the expense of the public. If there is no public school available that can meet the needs of a student, then the public school must pay for the student to attend private school. This must be approved by the school district first. Appropriate means that each student's learning needs and abilities are met. Children with disabilities are given access to specialized educational services, which are individually tailored to meet his needs. Families cannot take their child's educational experience for granted. It is up to them to monitor their child's progress and request appropriate placements and services if they feel their child is not benefiting from school.

The School

"Special Education and Related Services" under Public Law 94-142 means specially designed instruction tailored to meet the unique needs of the child with a disability.[37] This includes classroom instruction, physical education, home instruction and, when necessary, instruction in private schools, hospitals or institutions. Related services are defined as transportation and other developmental, corrective and supportive services necessary to enable the child to benefit. Examples of related services are physical, speech or occupational therapy, a psychologist, social worker, school nurse, or an aide. Parents should make sure and include every related service their child needs in their individualized education program (IEP). If the child is between the ages of birth and two, he may be enrolled in an early intervention program through an Individualized Family Service Plan (IFSP). It offers services to the family under Public Law 99-457.[38] This plan recognizes the needs of everyone in the family, not just the child with the special needs. Services included may help the parents, the siblings and the child with the disability.

Families must have their child evaluated to qualify to receive services at school. The school district is required to assess the child's needs and abilities every three years. The family's local neighborhood school can provide the initial assessment. Before a child's third birthday, the parents can contact the school and request a special education assessment. The school may refer the parents to the school nurse or the person who is in charge of giving the family the initial paperwork to fill out to begin the process. During the assessment or staffing, the child will be tested for social, academic, general intelligence or cognitive skills, language and communication ability, motor skills and emotional status. The school will also request a vision and hearing screening, as well as up-to-date immunizations and health records. The initial screening can last up to two hours. It is helpful if parents bring a snack or drink for their child since it can be a long process. When possible, both parents should attend all assessments. Parents will be asked for their input and observations. It is also helpful to come to staffings and Admissions, Review and Dismissal (ARD) meetings with a person who understands the special education process to help ensure that the child's needs are being met. This can be another parent from a support group who is familiar with the special education process or an advocate who has been hired by the family. Support groups, such as the National Parent Network, assist families by advocating for them in the school system. Many parents in this network have been trained in special courses which teach them how to advocate for education rights on behalf of the family. The courses are referred to as parent training information (PTI). Parent support groups which offer PTI's are located in every state. Families can contact the National Parent Network and request the name of their local network which offers parent training information. Being well-informed helps ensure that the child's education needs are met.

Many school districts have parent liaison centers which serve as a resource library and information center for special education parents and professionals. The Houston Independent School District Exceptional Education Parent Liaison Center is an example of one center which provides a link between parents and the school. Center administrators believe that each student requiring special education services deserves a knowledgeable team of parents and professionals working cooperatively to provide the best possible educational programs. It is the intention of the Exceptional Education Department to build trust and understanding among the members of the team through a series of ongoing services. It offers parent training workshops designed to inform parents of their positive involvement in the ARD/IEP decision-making process for their child. It offers training to community agencies to provide information on the ARD/IEP process, educational programs, advocacy and conflict resolution. Parent workshops are coordinated and support and training are provided for parents at ARD/IEP meetings with a Parent Liaison in attendance upon request. Parents can inquire at their local schools about a liaison center.

The beginning assessment can be an overwhelming experience for both the parents and the child. The child will be asked a variety of questions to access his cognitive, language and social skills. The parents will be asked to report what they know about those skills and fill out forms as well. At the end of the initial assessment, specialists will ask the family about their expectations or goals for their child. It is helpful if both parents discuss their goals

The School

and expectations from the school district. At the end of the initial assessment, parents will receive a general plan for their child which will be followed up in the Admissions, Review, and Dismissal Committee (ARD).

The purpose of a staffing is to decide what services the child needs according to test results and devise an Individualized Education Program (IEP). The results of the assessment should reinforce what the parents observe about their child at home. If the parents do not agree with the results of the tests, they can request that their child be allowed to take parts of the test over. If this is not possible, a third party can be called in to give the same test at the school district's expense. When the assessment is complete, it is discussed in the Admission, Review, and Dismissal Committee (ARD). The ARD is made up of teachers and other professionals who help the child with the disability. The committee is responsible for the admission, review of progress and dismissal of children to and from special education.

Suzanne Cuthbertson is the director of Arbor Pre-School, a private school for children with disabilities from ages birth to six. Suzanne advises that both parents visit a variety of schools to determine which one is most suitable to meet the needs of the child. They should consider the student-to-teacher ratio. In some programs there may be too many children assigned to one teacher. They need to ensure that the child will receive enough one-on-one attention to meet his needs. Parents should observe how the staff deals with the students and walk away feeling comfortable with what they see. Suzanne feels it is helpful for parents to observe other children in the classroom. It gives them a sense of hope for their own child.

During any evaluation phase, Suzanne reminds parents to remember that their child is being tested in a strange environment with people he does not know. The results should be taken with a "grain of salt." If parents do not agree with the results of the test, they can request the testing take place on another day and in another setting, such as the child's preschool setting, so the child feels more at ease. She feels testing in an unfamiliar setting is often misleading and can be inaccurate for students with disabilities.

Suzanne recommends that parents become familiar with child

development. It is important that they understand what they can expect from their child during different phases of development. It is useful to have this knowledge when formulating the child's Individualized Education Program (IEP). Arbor uses the Carolina Curriculum for Infants, Toddlers and Children with Special Needs, which is published by Paul Brookes, as a guide for their student's IEP's. Suzanne believes this curriculum is an appropriate resource for children who have disabilities. It provides practical skills which help teachers and parents break short- and long-term skills down into very specific categories. Suzanne feels that some schools do not break skills down far enough when formulating the IEP. If the skills suggested in the IEP are too vague, it is difficult to measure achievable and appropriate tasks. At Arbor, the staff updates each child's IEP once a month. Public school updates once a year. Suzanne suggests that parents request that their school district review goals at least every three months. They can be reviewed in parent-teacher conferences. The skills should be broken down with measurable, appropriate goals in writing. If the parents do not feel that their child is making progress, they should not wait until the next conference, as children with special needs cannot afford to lose any time. When the parent is uncomfortable with the lack of progress, he or she should call the school and discuss the matter with the appropriate teacher.

After the initial assessment is complete, the first ARD will be called. The family and an advocate, if the family has chosen one, come to school and meet with the team of specialists who will define the steps involved to meet the child's needs in the Individualized Education Program. The meeting should include a limited number of people who have a shared vision for the child.[39] Parents have the right to call an ARD when they feel they need to update or change the IEP.

Every IEP must include:

- A description of the student's present level of achievement.
- Short- and long-term goals.
- Specific educational services.
- Dates of services.

The School

- When services will begin and how long they will last.
- Methods to determine whether the student is meeting goals.
- The extent of mainstreaming in regular education.
- Vocational assessment by age fourteen or before the child enters high school.
- The extent, if any, of the child's participation will be in year-round services.
- Evaluation procedures.
- The schedules for determining the annual objectives and if they have been achieved and assistive technology needs.

Parents should document everything and keep all communications with the school in writing. All documents should be copied. When the school gives the child a classification or label, the parents must make sure that it is appropriate. It should be reviewed and updated as the child develops over time. In Texas, when a child is between the ages of three and five, they may be classified as "non-categorical early childhood eligibility" if parents request this. This applies to children receiving special education services who are too young to be given a diagnostic label for a specific disability.[40]

Each IEP category should include at least two or three objectives. A short-term instructional objective is a specific statement that addresses progress to be made within the next couple of months. It will take a specific action. The goal must be described in the steps it will take for the teacher to accomplish it. A short-term goal should answer what, when, who, how long, as well as the verbal instruction or reinforcement that will be used. All school personnel who will be working with the child must be aware of the objectives and work to achieve them.

An annual goal is a generalized statement of the progress desired, such as improving self-help skills, eliminating self-destructive behavior or improving understanding of basic math concepts. There can be several annual goals. One month before the annual review, the family should submit all of their reports to the committee and ask that all reports be sent to the family. This helps resolve any problems before the meeting takes place. The meeting should be attended by both parents and an advocate if the family chooses to bring one. All records and documents should be copied to ensure that everyone at the meeting has access.

The Carl D. Perkins Act mandates that vocational and transition planning take place for children with disabilities in public school at age fourteen. Parents will want to begin thinking about transition planning when their child is in elementary school. They may want to consider what types of skills the child will need to reach full potential. Transition planning should define goals which help the child develop personal, social and vocational skills.[41]

When the IEP is developed, it should include both functional and practical skills. When established early, it helps smooth the way for the adult service system to plan and provide services later on. The people involved in the IEP at this level may change. The family may want to include special education teachers, local vocational rehabilitation counselors, a transition planning teacher and a job coach when appropriate. A job coach will go on the job with the employee who has a disability and acts as a liaison between the employee and the supervisor. This team can help assess the student's level of vocational skills in the areas of work readiness, interests, social adjustment and aptitudes.

Transition planning can include internship opportunities in work settings. Parents should research their child's options early. There are waiting lists for most job training programs and workshops. A variety of employment programs are offered in many states. The school transition team should be able to identify these programs. One employment option is competitive employment in a regular work setting. A supported work model is job placement with on-the-job training and a job coach. An enclave is a job with full-time supervision. There are state-funded segregated work and vocational skill development programs. They include sheltered workshops and work activity centers. If none of the above options exist due to waiting lists or the unavailability of jobs, parents may have to find creative ways to invent placements for their child. They have to be prepared to call on employers themselves.

Transition planning involves preparing for college as well. The Adolescent Employment Readiness Center room helps teens with

The School

disabilities develop pre-employment skills. The Congress of Organizations of the Physically Handicapped, the Foundation for the Disabled and School to Work Transition Services all provide information for transition planning. The Heath Resource Center is a clearinghouse on postsecondary education for individuals with disabilities providing free publications, including *Financial Aid for Students with Disabilities, Vocational Rehabilitation Services—A Student Consumer's Guide,* and *How to Choose a College: Guide for the Student with a Disability. The Directory of College Facilities and Services for People with Disabilities,* written by James Thomas and Carol Thomas, can be found in the public library. It retails for $115. *Colleges That Enable: A Guide To Support Services Offered To Physically Challenged Students on 40 U.S. Campuses* by Prudence and Jason Tweed, can be found in book stores or the library. The Federal Student Financial Aid Program at the Office of Student Financial Assistance in Washington, D.C. can offer information about financial assistance if a state vocational rehabilitation agency has determined that the best preparation for a job for an individual with a disability is a college education. There are no special federal financial aid programs to assist individuals with disabilities to attend college unless they are referred by a vocational rehabilitation agency. The American Association of University Affiliated Programs for Persons with Developmental Disabilities can provide information to parents and students about related programs and services. The Association for Handicapped Students provides practical information for students who have disabilities. Many colleges and universities have programs and services which can assist people with disabilities.

Working Effectively With The School

Parents can help insure that their child's IEP is monitored and followed by becoming involved with the school on a regular basis. If they become a visible part of the working team, they have a better chance of overseeing their child's education. Parents can set up progress meetings with their child's teachers, even before the school year starts. It may be helpful for parents to request a copy of their child's school schedule to familiarize themselves as well as their child. Take the child to school before it starts and walk through the schedule by showing him his classrooms, the library, cafeteria and the playground. The orientation will help the child feel more comfortable. Let the child meet his teachers and specialists before school starts. Parents should give the child's teachers emergency numbers so they have quick access to either parent. It may be helpful on the first day of school, especially if it is a child's first experience, to stay close by. The parent may want to sit in the school office or go back to work and check in with the school during the day.

Some parents find it helpful to use a daily communication notebook with their child's teachers. The notebook serves as a way for the parent, specialists and teachers to give feedback about the child's progress. The notebook can include the IEP short-term goals and the tasks to master the goals. The days of the week and the staff members who will be working with the child can be listed. A space for comments is helpful to give the parents feedback about progress. The specialist working with the child can sign his or her name on the days he or she worked with the child and write down any comments he or she may have to help the child reach his goals. If problems arise, they can be mentioned in the notebook and taken care of early.

Parents can help their child have a positive experience in school by letting the teachers know they want to be part of the process. Parents can have a visible profile at school by volunteering to help in the classroom or becoming a room parent, coming in to read to the class, helping with holiday parties, taking the children on a field trip, educating the class about children with disabilities or educating the school administration about disabilities. There are many organizations that provide disability awareness training to schools. The National Easter Seal Society Communications Department offers a Friends Who Care Elementary School Awareness Program. The school receives hands-on lessons for the class as well as a videotape of students discussing what it is like to live with a disability. The Kids on the Block is a national organization made up of volunteers who go to schools and other community settings to teach people about disability awareness and social issues.

The School

They offer thirty-seven different programs and use puppets to teach. Dialing 1-800-368-KIDS will connect callers with their local Kids on the Block program. When teachers and administrators see a parent with a positive attitude and a desire to work cooperatively with them, it helps them work with the child in a positive way.

If problems do come up, it is best to start with the source. If it is a classroom issue, the parent can politely ask to speak with the teacher. Parents should approach the problem from an assertive point of view, without anger or threats, state the problem and suggest a possible solution. The goal is to get the teacher to listen and help come up with a solution. If there is no way to resolve the matter on this level, go to the next person in the administration and approach the situation with an assertive statement. If necessary, a parent can keep going up the ladder in the school administration. If it looks as if there will be no resolution, a last resort is requesting a Due Process Hearing, which is the parent's right under Public Law 94-142. It is something to consider when all else fails, as it can be very expensive and take a long time. A Due Process Hearing includes an evaluation of the child, an impartial hearing officer, an administrative appeal against the hearing officer's decision to a state commissioner or Department of Education, a complaint to a federal office for civil rights and the right to a final appeal to the civil courts.[42] Going to court requires the expertise of an attorney who specializes in disability laws. The family can find such an attorney through referrals from friends, a state or national disability agency, or through an advocacy agency. Some law schools provide legal advice at little or no cost to families. There are legal aid agencies which provide legal services at little cost. Support groups, such as the National Parent Network, can give referrals for legal service.

Mark Brown is an attorney for the Disability Rights Education Defense Fund (DREDF). He recommends that if parents have questions concerning their child's legal rights they call the Americans With Disabilities Hotline at 1-800-466-4232. They will be put in contact with an attorney who can answer questions about suspected rights violations. DREDF helps families secure the special education services guaranteed by state and federal laws. Parents can receive information and training about their children's rights under the law and support to help them ensure their children's educational needs are met. Representation in hearings and in court is also available.

The Council for Exceptional Children is dedicated to improving the educational outcome for people with disabilities. It can provide information about legal rights. The National Association of Protection and Advocacy, the American Bar Association Center and the Children's Defense Fund are other resources which can provide legal information pertaining to education rights.

School Experiences

Sara is a six-year-old student who has epilepsy. She attends regular elementary school in a class with children who have been mainstreamed. Some of the children have special needs. The school system has provided Sara with a part-time teacher assistant. Her parents hired an attorney to help them advocate for Sara's needs. The school district wanted Sara to ride the bus for children with disabilities instead of the regular school bus and the family had to fight to let her stay on the regular bus.

Matthew, who is eight, is hearing-impaired. His family had to fight his school district to get Matthew speech therapy.

Byron is a nine-year-old boy who has autism. His family has had to search for alternative ways to get Byron's educational needs met. They have learned a lot about the laws and realize the importance of understanding exactly how the IEP will meet Byron's needs.

Nine-year-old Brittany has cerebral palsy and attends a regular public grade school. She is in a self-contained classroom where she has occupational, physical and speech therapy. She participates in physical therapy, music, art, library and recess with the regular third-grade class. She takes special classes for reading, social studies and math. Her mother has hired an advocate to ensure that Brittany's needs are being met.

Betinna is a seven-year-old girl who is mentally retarded and has cerebral palsy. She is enrolled in a public elementary school and her teacher has encouraged the children in class to help Betinna when she needs it. The children help her get around school by taking her to the cafeteria, library and outside for recess. The children also take turns reading to Betinna. School has been a positive experience for Betinna and her mother credits her teacher, who encourages and motivates her to increase her self-help skills.

Jonathan is seven and has cerebral palsy. He attended special classes for kindergarten and early intervention. His parents felt that the expectation for Jonathan to learn in special education classes was too low. They felt that he was only expected to "knock pegs out of a pegboard." When they put him in regular classes, the expectations for learning were much higher and he did learn. He is not close to his peers in regard to his academic achievement, but he has grown and developed faster and farther than they ever dreamed. He has made many school friends who come over to their home even though his parents think they have little in common.

Allen is an eight-year-old boy who has autism. His mother is very disappointed in his educational experience. She feels that Allen's teachers are apathetic and the specialists have very little patience or coping skills. The principals do not want to become involved and instead redirect problems back to the superintendent of special education, who is already overworked. Allen does not see himself as having any special needs. When he is put in special education classes or on the special education bus, he gets angry, he swears, kicks and spits. When he is put in a regular classroom, he cannot handle the noise level. He spends a lot of the time in a storage closet they have set up as a room because the school is overcrowded.

Danielle is in second grade. She has cerebral palsy and a developmental delay. She attended intervention at ARC, the Association for Retarded Citizens, until she was two years old. She received services through the Easter Seal Society until she was four. Her elementary school provides life skills support classes for her.

Adrienne is a five-year-old girl who has cerebral palsy. She attends public preschool now and next year she will attend regular kindergarten with an aid. The school system has enabled her family to learn teaching techniques which facilitate Adrienne's communication. Adrienne likes school and is enrolled in a special early childhood class and is mainstreamed for part of the day. Adrienne's mother has conflicting feelings regarding a recent three-year comprehensive assessment through the school system's educational diagnostician. She felt that the results of the assessment were unfair to her daughter and the goals listed in her IEP are much too low for the amount of skills her daughter already has. The family was very offended by the vocational skills training suggestion the school district proposed, which included "how to clean, count money, etc." They felt that it was unfair to predict Adrienne's future and damage the family's hopes.

Aaron is a six-year-old boy who has autism but attends public school. His mother feels that his school experience has been "accepting and positive." Aaron attends a life skills class in the morning and regular first grade in the afternoon. His mother feels that he has wonderful teachers who encourage him.

Suggestions

- The quality of a child's educational experience depends on the working relationship between the school district, teachers, parents and related professionals. It is up to the parents to make sure the child's goals are being met.
- Find an advocate through a local parent support group, an attorney, or someone who understands the special educational process and take this person with you to the first assessment, staffing and Admissions, Review and Dismissal meetings.
- Understand what the IEP objectives are for your child and document everything.
- Become involved with the school and remain visible. Keep a communication notebook with the child's teachers and specialists as a method to monitor progress.
- Understand the laws and how they protect the rights of the child.

Chapter Nine

FUTURE PLANNING

Future planning begins when parents encourage their child to become as independent and self-reliant as possible. When children with disabilities are encouraged to reach their full potential, by providing them with opportunities in school, at home, in relationships, recreation and in the work place, parents are planning for the future. The levels of independence will vary according to the severity of the disability. Future planning helps to ensure that the person with the disability can live a comfortable life with adequate funds. Life planning is important for all people with mild to severe disabilities as it protects the person's future as well as the family estate. The aspects involved in planning should address what will happen to the person with the disability after the death of his parents, who will take responsibility for the person with the disability in caring for his needs, how financial needs will be met and who will provide other services that he may need.

Families must consider the cost-of-care liability, which is the right of the state providing care to someone with a disability to charge for their care and collect from that person's assets. If a person with a disability lives in a state-run facility, it requires payment for services. These services may be paid for through the state taking any personal assets from that person. If extended family or parents are planning to leave the person with the disability any inheritance, such as property, trust funds or any gifts in the form of money, the state can take any of these assets to pay for services if the person with the disability resides in a state-run facility.[43]

Richard Gorman is an estate planner for an estate planning

program for people with disabilities (EPPD). He recommends that parents disinherit their child who has a disability. In most states, with the exception of Louisiana and a few others, it is legal to disinherit a child. He recommends that parents set up a family trust which is sometimes considered a special needs trust. This enables the parents to put aside money for the person with the disability without jeopardizing government benefits. The money is distributed at the discretion of the trustee. The person with the disability has no direct involvement with the trust and a family trust will not be considered as income for that person. He will still be considered eligible for Social Security.

Richard suggests that parents educate relatives not to leave assets to the child with the disability because it can jeopardize chances of receiving government benefits. Their well-intentioned gift may be taken by the state to pay for the costs of living in a state-run facility. To receive government benefits, the person must be considered needy enough. If parents and other relatives leave property or money to the person with the disability, government benefits may be disqualified.

To determine if a person is eligible to receive Supplemental Security Income (SSI), the Social Security Administration evaluates if that person is unable to do any substantial gainful activity by reason of any medically deteminable physical or mental impairment which has lasted or can be expected to last for a continuous period of not less that twelve months. When a child reaches eighteen, the parents' income and resources are not used to determine eligibility. The eighteen-year-old may qualify for SSI if he has little or no income, is medically blind or disabled and does not work or works but earns less than the substantial gainful activity level. The family may apply for SSI several months before the person with the disability turns eighteen because the application process can take two to four months. They should apply at their local Social Security office and bring their child's birth certificate, Social Security number, medical records, physicians names and addresses and information about savings accounts, trust funds, insurance policies and property ownership. If these resources are over the limit, the child will be ineligible. The family should call beforehand and ask what specific records they should bring.

Future Planning

Documenting contacts at governmental agencies helps to ease the way through the maze of paperwork and people they will have to deal with.

Social Security Disability Insurance (SSDI) is money which has been paid into the Social Security System through payroll deductions. Disabled workers are entitled to these benefits. People who become disabled before the age of twenty-two may collect S.S.D.I. under a parent's account if the parent is retired, disabled or deceased.

Medicaid is a joint state and federal program that offers medical assistance to people who qualify for Supplemental Security Income. Medicare is a federal program that provides medical care to people who receive SSI.

The family will want to determine how well the person with the disability will be able to manage his own affairs. It is important to determine if the person will be capable of making decisions regarding future planning. The issue of mental competency and guardianship should be considered.

Insurance and retirement policies should be reviewed, making sure that adequate funding will be left to cover the needs of the person with the disability. They must remember to set up these policies without jeopardizing any government benefits for their child.

Parents should have a will, which should be reviewed periodically to make changes when necessary. It is important for the parents to express their wishes and intentions. If the parents have named their child with the disability as a beneficiary, they must remember that this may disqualify their child from receiving any government benefits. If the parents do not have a will and they die, the law requires that each child in the family share equally in the parents' estate.[44] If the family allows the state to divide their property, the person with the disability may be disqualified to receive any government benefits.

The family will want to consider living arrangements when applicable. These will vary in different communities. The type of living arrangement will depend on the person's level of independence skills and the amount of assistance needed. Choices include independent living, group homes, staffed apartments and rental assistance eligibility housing from United States Department of Housing and Urban Development (HUD). Applications must be made early to get on a waiting list for many of these options. Local health officials can provide more information about living arrangement options.

There are several professionals families can contact to begin planning. One choice is using a team approach with Estate Planning for Persons with Disabilities (EPPD). The team is made of family members, attorneys, financial planners, bank trust officers, life insurance underwriters and certified public accountants. The benefit to this type of planning is having all the professionals come together to give advice. There usually is a low, flat fee as opposed to each professional charging separate hourly rates.

The family may choose to put their own EPPD team together by hiring a team of experts, or one at a time as needed. The issues to address in each plan will vary according to the needs of the family as well as the needs of the person with the disability. When possible, it is important to involve the person with the disability so a mutual decision can be reached.

Suggestions

- Future Planning ensures that the person with the disability has the resources to live a comfortable life with adequate funds, protecting his future as well as the family's estate.

- Future Planning must consider the cost-of-care liability, government benefits and the ability of the person with the disability to make decisions. The family should examine insurance and retirement policies to make sure their is adequate coverage for the person with the disability without jeopardizing the person's ability to receive government benefits.

- Extended family members and parents do not want to disqualify government benefits for the person with the disability by leaving trust fund money, property or by naming the person as a beneficiary in a will. A special needs trust or family trust protects the person with the disability.

Future Planning

- Parents should draw up a will which protects the interests of the children and instructions for the division of their estate. Without a will, the state has the right to equally divide the estate among the children, which will jeopardize the government benefits for the person with the disability.
- Locate a team of experts to secure a future plan.

Chapter Ten

ADULTS WITH DISABILITIES LIVING MEANINGFUL LIVES:
SEVEN ADULTS SHARE THEIR EXPERIENCE

Caldwell's Story

Caldwell is thirty-eight, married and has two children. She is a second-grade teacher in Birmingham, Alabama. Because of Fetal Thalidomide Syndrome, she was born with two fingers on each hand, no foot on the right leg and two toes and a heel bone missing on her left foot. Her mother had ingested a form of thalidomide that was prescribed by her doctor for morning sickness during pregnancy.

Caldwell wears a shoe insert and a prosthesis. She is fully mobile and does not require any assistance. Her family had a vital role in helping her cope with her disability while growing up. They gave her love, encouragement and accepted her with a positive attitude. Her father and friends were her most supportive allies. Her parents treated her just like any other family member, for the most part. At times, Caldwell thought her family may have been a little more tolerant of her than they should have been. She felt that her parents sheltered and spoiled her and at the same time encouraged her independence. They allowed her to try whatever she wanted to try. They were never shocked or amazed when she accomplished something. She credits her parents for who she is today, but she used Helen Keller as her role model because she was an amazing woman who overcame more than most people ever face.

Caldwell's school experience was positive. She attended public school in a regular classroom. Her teachers had the same high expectations for her as the other students and were always available to give extra help, especially in physical education classes. She was treated with kindness at school and felt "special" in a good way.

Friends provide a source of support for Caldwell. She does not have friends who have disabilities. She shied away from the children with special needs; they made her feel "handicapped." The friends that she has made over the years treat her as totally normal, perhaps, she feels, with a little more respect and admiration because of her differences. One of the most difficult hurdles for her has been realizing that someone might not enjoy being with her because of her personality instead of her handicap. She has made some friends because of her disability that she would not have made otherwise.

Caldwell feels society responds more favorably toward people with special needs because people are more open to discussing their needs and limits. She feels any sense of shame over a disability has diminished and is viewed as an opportunity rather than a hindrance.

She chose to become a teacher of small children. With each new class, on the first day of school, she shares her disability with the students to avoid any uncomfortable feelings. Her choice of sports has not stopped her from using her sense of humor. She jokingly points out that water-skiing is a problem because she can't hang on to the bar and bowling is not her game. Neither of these really bother her, though she did always have a desire to be a fast runner.

Her spirituality has been "enhanced." She focuses on the inner self, not outward appearance. Caldwell does not feel that her disability has affected her sexuality. She explains that once she figured out whether to leave her leg on or take it off she felt comfortable. She feels totally accepted by her husband for who she is. They often joke that he must not be a leg man.

Caldwell's children just know her as "Mom." They seem proud of her artificial leg and big fingers now, although Caldwell worries that it could cause difficulty as her children get older. Motherhood has been a difficult transition for Caldwell. She says that going from being pampered to being the nurturer is hard and leaves her tired, which leads her to feeling sorry for herself.

Caldwell suggests that children understand that who they are is not determined by what they can do. They should try to understand that others are curious and everyone has a weak spot. She encourages them to go with the flow, do their best and enjoy life. Caldwell wants kids to know that the things that might seem important now will change. To parents raising children with special needs, she suggests that they always focus on what the child can do and stay positive. Appreciate who they are. Find their strengths and build upon them. Be available, but give them wings.

Caldwell feels that little children are afraid that a person with a disability is contagious or ill and may die. With adults, she feels that people have low expectations for people with special needs. She thinks that sometimes the "average Joe" needs to be more aware of his "specialness." Caldwell believes that people with disabilities are really in the limelight. She strongly discourages people from excessively catering to the needs of people with disabilities. Such catering can lead to dependence and lowered expectations.

Barbara's Story

Barbara is thirty-three, married and a mom. She works as a service provider for the deaf and serves as a curriculum coordinator at Central Christian Church Parents Day Out. She attended Gallaudet University, where she received her B.A. in Early Childhood Education and a Master's Degree in Education.

She has been profoundly deaf since eleven years of age due to repeated ear infections. Hearing impairments arise from many different causes, some of which are not known. People with hearing disabilities may have slight losses and hear a great deal or they may have great losses and hear very little. Some people use hearing aids. The word deaf means not being able to hear anything. To communicate, various forms of language are used: American Sign Language (ASL), Signed English or Cued Speech. Lipreading, speaking, writing, drawing pictures and gestures are some forms of expression which are sometimes used.

Adults with Disabilities Living Meaningful Lives

Barbara has a telecommunications device which enables deaf people and non-deaf people to talk to one another over the telephone lines using a small terminal with a screen and an abbreviated keyboard, something like a typewriter. She has a doorbell with lights and a baby cry signaler. She requires a sign language interpreter and does everything alone that doesn't require listening.

Her parents' faith and her school friends helped her cope. She attended public school beginning in junior high and was enrolled in regular classes. She says school was a positive experience but Barbara says if she could do it again, she'd want sign language interpreters. She believes that a school which is set up to meet the needs of children with disabilities is the best and thinks deaf children should go to deaf schools.

Over the years, societal attitudes have become more accepting of the deaf. Barbara believes the deaf are more accepted, especially with the successful protest to have a deaf president elected to Gallaudet University, the popularity of the Oscar-winning deaf actress Marlee Matlin and the selection of the first deaf Miss America, Heather Whitestone.

Barbara believes it is important for children with disabilities to have friends with special needs for support and to learn from one another. When she was growing up, she did not have friends with special needs and it wasn't until she attended Gallaudet University that she made deaf friends.

She majored in deaf education in school and her relationships are with deaf friends and/or people who can converse in sign. She married a deaf man and her children learned American Sign Language first to communicate with them.

The most difficult transition for Barbara was moving to Texas. She grew up in New York and Massachusetts where there were more programs for the deaf.

Barbara does not feel that there are enough services for young people preparing for their independence. She believes a lot of kids who are deaf or disabled are "stuck to Mommy or Daddy" and their Social Security checks that come in the mail. Barbara feels that it is vital for children to break away from parents and learn to go out on their own. She encourages them to learn to earn and budget their money, as well as to learn independent living skills.

Barbara advises young people to be themselves and fight for their rights as a deaf person. She encourages parents to expose their child to a variety of language modes and accept what the child chooses. She tells parents to avoid trying to make their child into something he is not and to remember that the child is deaf and will always be deaf. There is no miracle cure.

Barbara's practical advice to students is to "hang in there." She knows that there are a lot of people who struggle to prove their deafness is not a barrier. She encourages children to learn to communicate in public by writing notes or making gestures.

Barbara recommends that parents contact Gallaudet University for information for their children. She suggests reading books and watching movies about deaf culture. She recommends *Deaf Like Me, Growing in Silence, Children of a Lesser God* and *Your Name is Jonah*.

Brent's Story

Brent is a thirty-three-year-old language support specialist with Deaf Student Services, Texas State Technical College. He is married to Barbara and they have two children. He received his B.A. in social work from Gallaudet University.

Brent has been deaf since birth due to rubella. He is able to do anything alone that does not require hearing. While Brent was growing up, he credits his family with helping him cope with his disability.

He attended a residential day program at the Rochester School for the Deaf, a deaf-oriented program where they used sign language and finger-spelling. Brent prefers to see deaf children in deaf schools. He considers his school experience to be an excellent one.

Brent feels that he is treated well by both hearing and deaf peers. He senses that most people in the United States are becoming aware of people with disabilities with the help of the media and exposure to people with disabilities as effective role models.

His family attends a church that has interpreting services and they attend Sunday school class for deaf adults.

Brent advises school-age children to have friends with disabilities to provide peer support, which promotes feelings of cohesiveness and oneness. He tells them to focus on their own being and strengths to forge ahead to achieve their dreams. Brent would like to see more services for children and young adults with disabilities in schools instead of waiting until they graduate and get a job.

Robert's Story

Robert is a twenty-two-year-old single man who is a computer programmer who works from his home. He is a high-school graduate. He recently started Better Way BBS, a disability data base resource service.

Robert has cerebral palsy and requires attendant care, modified housing, a modified van with a lift and a van driver. He uses a motorized wheel chair and a walker. He wears long leg braces and can walk with support and he also crawls. In the shower, he uses a roll and a shower wheelchair. He sleeps in a hospital bed and needs help dressing, bathing, with meal preparation, cleaning and mobility.

Robert does not require help working on the computer, talking on the phone, going out in a cab and bookkeeping.

While he was growing up, his parents, friends and teachers helped him cope with his disability. He maintains a close relationship with his family. He lives at home and feels his mother has been supportive, yet somewhat overprotective. Robert's father is also supportive but sheltering. He feels that he was not treated as an equal member in his family because he needed extra help which took time and energy away from his other family members.

Robert's role models while growing up were his physical therapist and an attorney. The physical therapist always had a way to help him get the work done with new ideas. Robert attended public school and participated in the Individual Education Program. He was enrolled in special education classes for math, English and adaptive physical education. He was mainstreamed into seventh-grade speech and drama. In high school, a teacher helped him fight to become enrolled in her German class. She took extra time to test him during her break so that he could be tested orally. Robert's school was not wheelchair accessible. There were no hand railings in the bathrooms until he demanded that they be installed. Getting from one end of the building to another in a wheelchair required Robert to invent ways to maneuver.

Robert describes his friends as supportive. Some had disabilities. He feels that he was lucky to get one date in high school, taking a friend from the German Club to dinner. He had to bring his whole family along with him on the date, which cost $57.

The most difficult hurdles for Robert include finding good people for attendant care, going to school, finding a girlfriend, obtaining transportation, maintaining independence and obtaining financing for college.

Robert describes himself as a born-again Christian. He feels that his religion provides answers and comfort. He would someday like to marry someone with "a true heart" and have a family. He knows that he will not make as much money as he wants to because he must pay for his daily care. His Social Security checks help cover some of his expenses.

Robert advises parents raising children with special needs to make life as normal as possible. He urges children keep a positive attitude and find one thing they like to do and do it. For high-school students he recommends preparing early for college or work.

Randy's Story

Randy is thirty-seven, single and an athlete. He competes internationally in tennis tournaments and basketball. He and some friends formed a basketball team for athletes in wheelchairs. He plays the guitar, uses a computer, rides a bike and goes fishing. He is a motivational speaker and educates children about how important it is to see a person, not just a wheelchair. He is employed as an educational representative for Quickie Designs, Inc. and has a BBS in Marketing.

At age sixteen, Randy was in a car accident and was diagnosed as T12 traumatic paraplegic. Randy credits progressive rehabilitation, the tough love of his family and recreation with helping him cope with his disability. He received a great deal of support from his mother and a peer group with similar specific disabilities. His family treated him like a family member, not a disabled family member.

Randy uses adaptive driving equipment and some medical equipment, including a wheelchair. He does not require help with anything relating to his disability, but he requires a great deal of help pertaining to his life.

He attended public school and found it very difficult, as he felt he had trouble fitting in. He was enrolled in regular classes and required no special education. He felt he was treated okay by most school children, although there was some teasing. His school was not accessible, which was discouraging. He had friends with similar disabilities and found it helpful because it provided peer support.

Randy feels it is more difficult to be a male with a disability because of chivalry, like wanting to open a door for a woman and not being able to do so. He says he is treated like any disabled person in society; and that depends on the person.

The most difficult hurdle for Randy has been accepting himself as an equal member of society, which he finds patronizing. He feels the most common misconception regarding people with physical disabilities is that they are underestimated intellectually. He has seen attitude changes, with more acceptance, awareness and education.

Randy feels his disability has enhanced professional, spiritual and emotional aspects of his life, but has inhibited his intimate relationships. His disability has taught him that "we are all God's children, all of us." He wishes this could be realized by more people. He has had some amazing experiences, suffered incredible losses, gained intimate friends and reaped grateful rewards from being "disabled."

Randy advises parents raising children with special needs to force themselves to incorporate tough love, because enabling children is dangerous. He strongly believes that the family should integrate the person with the disability into their lifestyle. He recommends that high-school students hang on and get involved in the things they did before they became disabled. Being part of a group or clique is important during the teenage years. Randy tells children to remember that they are "okay." A disability can be used as an advantage, he says. Pursue your own dreams.

Lynn's Story

Lynn is a fifty-seven-year-old author and retired legal secretary. She is married and has three grown children. She was diagnosed with lupus and rheumatoid arthritis. Lupus is a chronic, progressive, usually ulcerating skin disease. It is thought to be an autoimmune disorder. Rheumatoid arthritis is a chronic systemic disease characterized by inflammatory changes in joints and related structures that result in crippling deformity.

Lynn now wears a fixed-ankle brace on her left leg. She experiences weakness, fatigue and depression. She has deteriorating joints in her right ankle, right hip, neck and lower back. This limits the distances she can walk. She requires help with lifting, opening heavy doors and going up and down stairs. She can do almost anything if it isn't a long-term or long-walking project. She tires easily and has to rest.

Dealing with a newly-acquired disability at middle-age has been a difficult transition in Lynn's life. Her family and friends have provided her with support. She knows that she feels differently about herself now. She feels that she is not as confident, not as pretty or sexy, not "normal," but since she has only had the brace a few months, she doesn't know how much is her perception. She feels men don't see her as a woman anymore, kids stare and sometimes she thinks she sees pity in people's eyes. Lynn has always had doors opened for her in the past and had people smile at her when as she passed by. They still do, but she notices the glances at her brace. She asks herself if she is paranoid.

The relationship with her family has been very positive for the most part. Lynn has one daughter who has very little patience with any complaints from her. She is upbeat, overcomes obstacles with determination, hard work and perseverance, and thinks everyone should. Of course, Lynn thinks that she's right. Her daughter tells Lynn that she should never mention the brace or her illness and no one else will bring it up. But, Lynn feels like that is ignoring the obvious. Lynn's friends want to know what happened. Once she gets past the newness of it all, Lynn feels that maybe she can ignore it better. Her son acknowledges it, but doesn't seem to react in any noticeably different way. He's generally very stable as far as relationships go. Lynn's other daughter hasn't seen the brace, but on the telephone she wants to know all about it, how it feels, and how Lynn feels. All of her children worked with disabled kids when they were in high school. Lynn feels that her family is probably more able than most to accept her disability.

Lynn says one of the most difficult hurdle for her is realizing all the "I'll never-be-able-to's" of her life: dance, wear high-heels, hike, bicycle, roller-blade—many things she says she would never do anyway, but she feels as if they've been taken away from her. But the biggest hurdle is never feeling really sexy. Lynn has been married to the same man for forty years. It doesn't bother him. He still loves her and still thinks she is sexy. They still make love but Lynn has to initiate it. He is afraid the she is in pain or not feeling "up to it" and he doesn't want to pressure her. Lynn appreciates his concern, but it is hard for her to believe he wants her when she has to start it.

Lynn had to quit working full time. She can't dance, but writing is a primary leisure activity which she completes in shorter time spans. Her spirituality helps her make it through each day. She trusts that God will help. She does not believe the "He did it" to her but that He gives her courage, faith and strength to keep going.

The most difficult transition for Lynn has been figuring out who she is now and what that means. She says the most common misunderstanding about people with disabilities is that they are their disability.

Lex's Story

Lex is a forty-six-year-old married man, a professor of Physical Medicine and Rehabilitation at Baylor College of Medicine in Houston. He is the senior vice-president of research at the Texas Institute for Rehabilitation and Research (TIRR).

In 1967, when Lex was a freshman at Oklahoma State University, he was involved in an automobile accident. He and four other students were out late drinking and driving. They were involved in a head-on collision with another car full of students. All of them were rushed to the hospital. Lex was the last one to be examined because he had no apparent cuts and bruises, but could not move. He was diagnosed with a spinal cord injury, C-5 quadriplegia. He spent five weeks on the orthopedic floor of the hospital after a laminectomy and fusion. A laminectomy is the excision of a vertebral posterior arch. He spent three more months at TIRR for rehabilitation.

He is paralyzed from his shoulders down. He has no functional use of his legs and limited use of his arms. He uses an orthotic device which is connected to his arm which enables him to write and use the computer. His computer has a microphone and speech dictation ability, which allows him to write. He uses a powered wheelchair for mobility unless he is traveling. He prefers to use a manual wheelchair on airplanes, since it gets thrown around in baggage compartments. When Lex flies, he can bring his wheelchair into the first row of seats in first class on a 747 aircraft without having to use an aisle chair to transfer from. If he flies on planes which are not 747s, he uses an aisle chair to transfer from the wheelchair to his seat. Lex is unable to drive and uses public transportation.

Lex has had a personal care attendant since 1972. They have a mutual agreement to help each other out. Mack's disability was the result of a brain injury and it left him with some memory and cognition loss. Since Lex has an undergraduate degree in psychology, he agreed to help Mack with his cognitive deficit if Mack agreed to be his personal care attendant. They have been together since then.

The summer after Lex had his accident and rehabilitation, he wanted to return to his studies at college. In rehabilitation, he was told that whatever he was planning on doing before the accident would be attainable again, but from a wheelchair. He applied to Oral Roberts University to continue with his studies. He chose this university for a variety of reasons. He felt that since it was a relatively new university, with modern architecture, it would be a barrier-free environment with high-quality audiovisual equipment and technology. He also chose the school because of the faculty. He received a letter stating that his admission had been denied. Lex called the Dean of Admissions thinking they had made a mistake. He asked the Dean if he had read about his qualifications: valedictorian in high school, ranking in the top five percent in the SAT, earning a Regent scholarship that paid for part of his tuition, being captain of the golf team and getting a letter of recommendation from his minister. The Dean replied that he had read about all of the qualifications, but Lex could not be admitted to ORU because his application stated that he used a wheelchair. The Dean told Lex that he would be an imposition to the students and faculty. This was one of the most difficult hurdles Lex has had to face.

Lex decided to attend The University of Tulsa, where he received a warm welcome by the Dean of Students who asked how the university could meet his needs and make the necessary accommodations. He graduated in three and one half years with a degree in psychology and pursued a Master's Degree in Social Psychology at the University of Houston.

In 1984, he was asked to be a co-author of "Toward Independence," a report that detailed eleven recommendations to Congress regarding the rights of people with disabilities. This report was presented to President Reagan in 1986. In 1988, Lex became involved with "On the Threshold of Independence," a published piece of legislation which served as a report card of the first eleven recommendations. This became what is known today as The American Disabilities Act (ADA). The first of the eleven principles is considered to be a true Bill of Rights for people with disabilities. In July of 1990, the ADA was passed.

When asked how he felt about having played such an important role in the ADA, Lex replied, "I was at the right place at the right time. It was a coincidence. If it hadn't have been me, it would have been someone else. It was passed because of the millions of people living with discrimination."

Lex has seen changes since that time. He jokes that there are a lot more parking spaces now. Attitudes have changed a great deal. He feels that the media has helped people become aware of people with disabilities. Twenty years ago, people with disabilities were not seen out in public, in jobs, the grocery store, the theaters. Lex feels that the media has helped to "normalize" people with disabilities. In the not-too-distant future, Lex sees people with disabilities advancing with new technology, training and assistance.

Lex says his personal experience with discrimination depends upon the nature of the people and place. At airports, when someone is pushing his wheelchair, people will direct their conversation to the attendant, not Lex. In restaurants, it has been know to happen that Lex pays the bill with his credit card or cash and the waiter brings the receipt or change to another person seated at the table. He is quick to point out that he doesn't let these events frustrate him. He doesn't feel compelled to educate people about these small annoyances. He chooses to focus his energy educating people in a bigger way.

After his accident, both parents were supportive. His mother became his attendant. She never complained about it and tried to help him with physical assistance. She compared it to when he was an infant. His father was a bit shy about the personal care. He felt hurt and frightened after Lex had his accident. The physicians at the hospital asked his mother if they wanted Lex to live or die. His mother asked if he would be able to use his head and the physician replied, "Yes." His mother told the doctors to do anything they could to keep him alive. His father bodily carried Lex to his first advocacy meeting, while Lex bitterly cried that his dad was violating his personal rights.

In 1976, Lex met a woman whom he married in 1978. They met at TIRR and the University of Houston. They were both involved in the Coalition For Barrier Free Living. His wife has a disability which resulted from coma. She has paraplegia and uses a wheelchair. Together, they are raising his wife's four-year-old grandson, Trey. Lex describes Trey as a sensitive child. He tells his grandfather that he would like to trade with him sometime. He would like to use the wheelchair, while Lex walks. Sometimes Trey throws the ball real far just so Lex can't reach it, acting like a typical four-year-old.

Lex at times wishes that he could play the trumpet like he used to. When he feels like that, he listens to Herb Alpert instead.

He wishes that he could swim and play golf. But instead he "surfs the Internet." He figures that there just isn't enough time to do everything. He has traveled around the world. He doesn't know if his life would have enabled him or taken him in the direction he has chosen after his accident. He knows that he is only one of fifteen people in wheelchairs who have visited the Great Wall of China.

He says children with disabilities have to imagine what they want to do and then find the resources to do that. Role models are important. When Lex was growing up, his role model was Mickey Mantle. He even has his autograph. There were very few people with disabilities who could serve as role models when Lex was growing up, but things are different today. Lex says, "If someone tells you that you can't do something, use that as your motivation to achieve your goals."

To parents raising children with disabilities, Lex encourages them to be strong advocates for their children. "Parent Power" is more effective than consumer power. He reminds parents not to take benefits for granted. Despite improvements in programs and services, children still need support, guidance and encouragement. Lex recommends Centers for Independent Living as support centers for families. There are two hundred centers throughout the United States which are understaffed and underutilized. With an investment in time and money, these centers could serve as meaningful meeting places.

Jane's Story

Jane is a thirty-four-year-old married woman with a three-year-old son. She is a physical therapist employed at a children's hospital. She has a B.S. Degree in physical therapy from the University of Texas Medical Branch, Galveston, and a Master's Degree in Health Administration from Southwest Texas State University.

She has cerebral palsy and spastic diplegia, which affects her balance and movement in her legs. It is difficult for her to walk stairs without side railings to hold onto for support. She cannot climb on top of chairs to hang blinds. Her mobility is not affected.

She requires some help with balance tasks. If she has to carry her son over long distances or over difficult terrain, she knows to plan ahead and pack a stroller. If she feels unbalanced, she takes her child by the hand to steady herself. Planning ahead is something Jane does if she knows she is going to a place such as a stadium or an arena where there may be an absence of railings to hold onto when climbing stairs. She always tries to purchase ground-level tickets. Older buildings pose a hazard due to their inaccessibility. If Jane is alone, older buildings are barriers due to stairs without rails. Driving on freeways presents a challenge as well. Jane avoids high traffic at high speed due to difficulty coordinating eyes, hands and feet.

If Jane needs help, she is not shy about asking for it. She says she has to be brave. She has been known to ask strangers if she could borrow their arm for thirty seconds, if she feels the need for balance. She relates a funny story about a day in a department store when her toddler son ran away from her up a flight of stairs. She grabbed a stranger by the arm and said, "That's my son up there, could you go and get him for me?" She says she is never silent when she needs help.

Jane began preschool at two years of age. She attended a Montessori program and was very bright and verbal. Her parents recognized that she needed the stimulation from school early on. Jane's parents were instrumental in mainstreaming her into a regular school program before mainstreaming existed. On the first day of registration, her parents went alone. They told the school officials that Jane was home sick with the chicken pox. The truth was, her parents were afraid if the school administrators saw Jane had a physical disability, they would assume she was mentally impaired as well. In the days prior to inclusion, children with special needs ended up in inappropriate special education classes. Her parents knew that once Jane was enrolled in a regular education program, she would succeed. By the time Jane had taken her first exam, it was too late for the teacher to think she should be enrolled in special education. She received a perfect score.

Jane was the only child with a disability in elementary school. She describes those years as tough, since much of the emphasis was on physical performance. She couldn't play Red Rover or hit the ball in baseball. If she were on a team and they would lose, the children would tease her. Some would physically abuse her by hitting her and knocking her down. It happened most often at recess or free play while the teachers were not present. She felt that some of the children resented her.

She had surgery at age eight to help straighten her legs. She wore bilateral metal leg braces until she was fourteen years old. She hated the braces. They were ugly, stained and made her walk slower. People paid a lot of attention to them and some teachers were afraid and treated her like a handicapped person.

One of the positive elements during Jane's early education years was that school reinforced her good grades. This made her believe in herself. She was enrolled in accelerated classes. Her parents provided a wide variety of social settings for Jane, which increased her confidence as well. They exposed her to travel and many of their friends, which enabled Jane to become comfortable with people and new settings. Her parents' friends asked her questions about her legs, which gave Jane the chance to openly discuss her disability. They would often tell Jane that she was so brave and so well-adjusted, which reinforced her confidence.

Junior high school marked another turning point. She felt more respected. She became a candy-striper at a local hospital which gave her further exposure and enhanced her confidence. Her self-esteem was high as she felt increasingly more comfortable in social situations. At age fourteen, she and her friends built a bonfire and burned the shoestring laces which held her braces together. It was a day of triumph for Jane. She never wore braces again.

At sixteen, she began dating and babysitting. She also took an extended trip to Europe and continued traveling throughout the country. She credits these adventures with giving her more practice in a variety of settings, which helped build her confidence.

When it was time for college, she decided to move to another state and begin her journey toward independence.

During Jane's lifetime, she has seen changes in societal attitudes regarding people with disabilities. People with disabilities have both a job and a place in society now. Education and recreation have changed to include everyone now and that is new. Two of the things that seem to remain the same are ignorance and prejudice.

One of the most difficult hurdles for Jane happened during college. She was told by clinical physical therapy instructors that she shouldn't become a physical therapist due to her physical disability. Jane chose to ignore this advice and passed her physical therapy boards with flying colors. She chose this field because she had always been fascinated with the medical field and wanted to work with children. Her job enables her to give hope and inspiration to children and families with special needs.

A common misconception regarding people with physical disabilities, according to Jane, is that they are mentally impaired or unable to function as others do.

Since graduate school, Jane has married a man who is nondisabled. She has one son. She tells a funny story about buying her wedding dress.

"I bought my wedding gown in one day. It took four days to find the right shoes."

Shoes have always been a problem due to the support they must provide for balance and stability. While she was growing up, she had a special aunt who she called her shoe aunt. Whenever Jane found a pair of good supportive shoes, her aunt would buy her nine pairs of the same shoe. Jane wished that all her dresses could be like her wedding gown. It weighed her down and helped her balance.

Jane's advice to parents raising children with special needs is to build your child up from the inside and let them go as far as they can. Her parents allowed her to do everything.

She advises teenagers to determine their purpose in life, have a mission and keep self-esteem high. Goals and high expectations are important. She says they should take school seriously and carve out a learning experience, find friends and not beat their heads against the wall because of the unenlightened. You will become the manager of your care, she says. Know your resources.

"Plan early for college. Connect up with university disability services. If you require adaptations or attendant care, ask for it. Talk, approach and teach people about yourself. Above all, remember, you are going to survive," Jane says.

She wouldn't want to be an ordinary person. Jane feels that her life has been enriched and she takes nothing for granted.

Chapter Eleven

SINGLE PARENTS

The diagnosis of a disability, chronic illness and the increase in demands which often accompany additional disabilities or complications as the child reaches or does not reach milestones increase any family's stress level. Unexpected life events call upon family members to redefine their roles, expectations, and eventually restructure their family system.[45] How a family restructures depends upon how each partner responds emotionally to the unexpected situation, how close the relationship was before the event and the severity of the situation. Many factors affect the health of a marriage. In some relationships, communication may fail and pull partners apart. In other relationships, unresolved conflicts may arise out of the sheer exhaustion resulting from new caretaking demands. Each individual's level of maturity and coping skills in dealing with a painful situation may differ. The couple will no doubt have the increased financial pressure of additional medical bills. The pressure could be heightened if one partner is no longer able to continue working to provide for the child's needs at various therapies, special schools and medical appointments. The quality of the spousal relationship before the diagnosis may have been poor. The stress of raising other children enters into the situation. The parents may not have access to social support from friends, family or community. One partner may be managing more of the daily care of the child who has the disability and thus becomes the information resource. This creates extra stress and widens the communication gap between the parents.[46]

The family may have neither the strength nor the stability to carry on as a single unit. Some marriages simply cannot survive. The parents may feel a need to separate.

Single parents raising children with special needs face a great challenge. They have complex financial concerns. Emotional issues related to the absence of a partner and the assessment of their role as a single parent raising a child who has special needs can be draining. The single parent faces greater parenting responsibilities. He or she must meet the basic demands of supplying food, clothing and a home for the family. The parent must continue to meet the medical, social, educational and future needs of all the children in the family. All of these considerations must be faced in addition to dealing with the parent's own needs.

If there has been a divorce, both parents' grief for the loss of their marriage which is magnified by the feelings of sorrow over the child's disability. The intense emotional climate which has already been in existence is heightened during the period of separation and divorce. The parents face the pressures of dividing up property and relocating. They face loneliness and the lack of intimacy with a mate.

Living in separate places puts additional stress on the parents to communicate the needs of the child as well as dividing up tasks to meet the child's needs. One partner may not follow up with intended care such as therapy appointments or giving the child medications. The parents may have different expectations of one another and of their children. They may disagree about parenting styles. One parent may feel that the partner who has primary custody of the child with the disability is overprotecting that child. This partner may not agree with how the other manages the professional help his or her child receives. The parent may disagree with the amount or types of therapies, the type of school program which has been selected or the medical management decisions which have been made by the other parent.

The communication which is already strained then becomes more complicated and disjointed. Heated conversations may erupt between the former partners revolving around one parent feeling the burden of care because the other parent is not doing his or her fair share. The parent who makes daily decisions for the care of the child who has the disability may have to do so alone due to the inaccessibility of the other parent. This creates more stress. This parent has no one with whom to discuss daily management and future planning for the child. This parent must rely on his or her own judgement under an often confusing barrage of information and choices. Once decisions have been made and discussed between both parents, there may be further questions that the caretaker must answer when justifying the choices to the non-caretaker. This creates feelings of anger and frustration for both parents. The parent who makes most decisions feels angry that the other parent is unavailable to be there but demands to know why certain decisions were made without his or her consent or input. When lines of communication are left open and continually updated, it helps to smooth over miscommunication and negative feelings. The parents may decide to communicate over the telephone, by mail or in person. It is best to keep their issues separate from those of the children.

Managing the other children in the family and dividing responsibilities between parents will create stress. The parents have to find time to meet all the children's needs by providing quality time with each child. Some parents may be unavailable or unwilling to commit to the family unit once they separate. Others will find the time to help with co-parenting.

One parent may have to relocate. If it is the caretaking parent, he or she has to secure new therapists, physicians, financial benefits, and retell the child's history to new professionals who will be involved with his or her care. A change in socioeconomic status of the parent who has the sole responsiblity for the child or children may occur. This parent may have to reside in a place that is more affordable but less pleasing and suitable. The caretaking parent may experience a change in his or her occupational status which adds to the existing pressures. If the parents relied upon one another to help balance the needs of the children and their respective jobs before the separation, the caretaking parent is left alone to manage this complex job. This parent may have to create new options so that he or she can meet the new demands. Some single parents may work part-time, full-time, and some may choose to stay home with the children. Securing childcare or respite care so the parent can be employed is an overwhelming task. When a child with a disability has special health or medical concerns, it can be frightening for the caretaking parent to trust another to meet that child's needs.

Single parents find it difficult to find time alone. Single parents are often exhausted from extra responsibilities. They find it difficult to locate good babysitters or respite care for a child who may require extra assistance due to his or her disability. Finding someone to trust if there is not a family member or a reliable sitter makes it more difficult for the single parent to have a social life outside the family. Trusting a stranger to take care of a child who has special needs is compounded by issues of not knowing if the child will be taken care of properly.

Dating, remarriage and the blending of families can create extra stress both positive and negative. Adding a supportive partner can help the parent meet his or her social and intimacy needs. A partner can also provide love, comfort and an added dimension of support for the family unit. Blending families requires understanding, patience and education. The new partner should have accurate information regarding the child who has a disability so he or she understands the implications involved.

Supportive extended family members, support groups and friends can also help alleviate some of the isolation the single parent faces.

One Single Mother's Experience

Anita is the single parent of one son. Alec is two years old and he was diagnosed at four months with a developmental delay. Anita suspects that her son has cerebral palsy but it is too early to tell. Alec spent his first eight days of life in the intensive care unit of the hospital, due to complications. At eight months of age, Alec required surgery. Alec's father left Anita after the surgery. Anita felt that he left them because he could not cope with Alec's situation. He was afraid that his son would die. Anita felt that her ex-husband never changed his expectations about her or Alec after the diagnosis had been made. He wanted things to be the same as before. He had been away from the family until very recently after the death of his mother. He helps with some of the finances for Alec's private school. He does not help with any of Alec's other needs. Occasionally, he watches his son so his ex-wife can make a short trip to the grocery store alone. They have the same problems they had before. They disagree about decisions made for Alec. Anita feels that she has had to make every major decision for Alec alone and afterward she is treated unfairly by her ex-husband. He questions her decisions, does not provide support and then does not want to discuss the situation. Their communication gap continues to widen.

One of the most difficult hurdles for Anita has been finding time for herself. She knows how important it is to do this. It is a struggle for her to trust her respite caretaker or a babysitter. She does go out occasionally, but not as often as she would like. It is expensive for her to do this and often takes a lot of preparation. She has no family support, so she must rely on near strangers. Anita knows that eventually she will have to find someone reliable and trustworthy to care for Alec since she plans on going back to work. She does not like depending on government assistance. For now, she gives the sitter lots of emergency information. She also carries a pager as does her ex-husband. If Anita is needed, the sitter can contact her right away.

After the separation, Anita and Alec had to move from a house in a nice neighborhood to an apartment complex filled with people drinking alcohol and selling drugs. They tried to live in a different city for a short time. Anita found this overwhelming. She had to retell Alec's story over and over to various new professionals. They all had different opinions about Alec. Hooking up with new therapists and medical professionals was very stressful for Anita. She made the decision to move back to the same city and to the same professionals who treated Alec initially. Her socioeconomic level declined. She compared herself to a "homeless person." She applied for Aid to Families with Dependent Children (AFDC) and she used up her savings to pay for the deposit on the apartment.

Anita's financial concerns include paying for everyday needs such as food and clothes and formula for Alec. She also has the extra financial responsibility of providing for her son's medical needs. He receives occupational therapy, physical therapy, and will eventually need speech therapy. Anita organizes all of her son's medical appointments. She was approved to receive SSI and food stamps. She had a job as a teacher's assistant at a day school but could not maintain a normal life. Alec was accepted at a private special needs school and Anita is responsible for transporting him back and forth. She made the decision to give up her job so she would be able to meet her son's needs. Her life revolves around Alec's needs for the present time. She is investigating public school options so that she will be able to someday reenter the work force.

Anita tries to stay optimistic. This helps her to move forward. She decided early on that she had a choice about her life with Alec. She could either do all she could for him to make sure that he has as normal a life as possible or she could do nothing and stay depressed. She lives one day at a time. She takes care of what she can each day and then there is tomorrow to take care of the new demands. She reads every available resource she can find to make sure that Alec is receiving what he is entitled to receive. She gathers information from the medical library and resource services. Anita believes in getting several opinions at a time so that she is sure that the diagnosis is accurate and the treatment meets her son's needs. She has a very strong spiritual belief and this helps her find guidance. She hopes to someday remarry and misses intimacy with a mate. Anita hopes to provide a happy and normal life for Alec and help him reach his potential. She does not want people to look at her son with pity. She finds societal perceptions most difficult to accept. Anita feels that everyone should be treated as a gift, not as "different" or not fitting in.

Suggestions

- Single parents face greater challenges to provide for the needs of the family. Parents should investigate every available resource which they are entitled to receive for their child.
- If relocating, single parents must be aware of the added stress this may cause in locating medical services as well as retelling their child's history to strangers.

Single Parents

- Locate a babysitter or respite care-worker to take time out alone. Provide every available emergency number to the caretaker.
- To deal with isolation, contact a local support group or stay in touch with friends and extended family members.
- Keep lines of communication with ex-spouse open when possible by writing letters, making telephone calls, and meeting in person to discuss the decisions regarding the children together. Ask ex-spouse to help share responsibilities.

Chapter Twelve

ALTERNATIVE CARE

Relinquishing the care of a child who has a disability may be an option for some families. This may occur at birth after a diagnosis has been determined, or later as the child grows and the parents feel that they are unable to meet the demands in the most beneficial way for the child.

There are many adoption agencies throughout the country that place children who have special needs. Many couples who either cannot conceive a child of their own, or others who have an interest in caring for children with disabilities open up options for parents who determine that adoption may be the best solution for them.

If parents have doubts about placing their child up for adoption, they can contact an adoption agency about temporarily placing their child in foster care while they make their final decision.[47] During this time they can find out about the adoptive parents from the agency. They can also contact local support groups and agencies which deal with the specific diagnosis of their child. They may want to contact other parents who have been in similar situations and ask them questions. Some things to consider may include how other families made the decision to keep their babies with the disabilities and how life has been for them. They may also want to interview families who have chosen to give their babies up for adoption and how they have dealt with this.

Up with Down Syndrome Foundation is a nonprofit agency which services families who have special needs. They provide respite care, foster care, hospice care and placement for adoption as well as information about the process of adoption. The National Adoption Information Clearinghouse provides information to parents who want to learn about the process of adoption and how to begin the proceedings. The Spina Bifida Association and the Down Syndrome Congress can provide adoption information as well. Other information can be found through local synogogues, churches, social and family services as well as through the Department of Health and Rehabilitative Services.

Residential placement is another option if the family determines that this type of care is the best solution for their child and for their family. As the child grows, needs change and demands for care may increase as well. The parents are aging and may not have the assistance and support of extended family anymore, if ever. They may be unable to take care of the child. If the child's disability is severe and the parent is aged, or lives alone as a single parent, then looking into options early on will be important to ensure that the child's needs will be met in the future. Parents may feel worn down by the daily care and it may be very difficult to survive as a family due to the severity of the disability and the strain placed on the family. They may be financially and emotionally burdened beyond what they feel they can manage. For some families to survive, they admit that the strain is too much for them to handle. They decide over time that a residential placement may be the best alternative. Parents who struggle with this often feel a tremendous amount of guilt. Seeking out a professional counselor who has experience with families facing these issues can be helpful when making this decision.

There are a variety of institutional or residential settings. They should all be examined early on because of waiting lists. Visits to all possible locations should be made early by family members to get a feel for the right environment. There are large and small facilities as well as group homes and supervised apartments. Families can locate possible options through local social service agencies, hospitals, physicians and support groups. The American Network of Community Resources and Options known as ANCOR and the National Association of Private Residential Facilities for the Mentally Retarded provide information about private facilities.

The Directory for Exceptional Children provides information about private and public facilities. The National Association of Private Schools for Exceptional Children also gives information regarding placements.

GLOSSARY

advocacy: The act of supporting or promoting a cause. Speaking out.

American Sign Language: Special grammatical structured unspoken language with its own syntax which allows for the exchange of ideas on many levels.

ARD Committee (Admissions, Review and Dismissal Committee): The committee is made up of teachers and other professionals. It is responsible for the admission, review and dismissal of children to and from the special education program.

assessment: The process of determining a child's strengths and weaknesses. It includes testing and observations performed by a team of professionals and parents. It is usually used to determine special education needs. The term is sometimes called an evaluation.

augmentative and alternative communication (AAC): A form of communication used by nonverbal children; often a device operated with eye blinks or by touch. It is the use of non-speech techniques such as signs, gestures or pictures to supplement speech abilities.

autism: A biological disorder characterized by an inability to process and use language, social and sensory information in a normal way.

cerebral palsy: A term used to describe the group of disorders that affect the way a child's muscles move.

cleft palate: A birth defect caused by the failure of the roof of the mouth (palate) to fuse properly, resulting in an opening on the roof of the mouth that leads to the nasal cavity.

congenital: Present at birth.

cognition: The ability to know and understand the environment.

cost-of-care liability: The right of a state providing care to someone with disabilities to charge for the care and to collect from that person's assets.

developmental delay: A delay in achieving certain skills when expected. It is usually associated with infants and children under the age of seven.

developmental disability: A severe, chronic, mental or physical impairment that occurs before the person reaches age twenty-two, the developmental years. It substantially limits the person's ability in such things as self-care, language, learning, physical mobility, self-direction, ability to live independently or economic self-sufficiency.

down syndrome: The most common chromosomal disorder occurring in one out of every 800 births. It is the major known genetic cause of mental retardation. The degree of mental retardation varies from mild to moderate. People with down syndrome are very capable of learning.

due process hearing: Part of the procedure established to protect the rights of parents and special needs children under Public Law 94-142.

epilepsy: A recurrent condition in which abnormal, electrical discharges in the brain cause seizures.

estate planning: Formal, written arrangements for handling the possessions and assets of people after they have died.

Glossary

free appropriate public education: The basic right to special education provided at public expense. This right is guaranteed by Public Law 94-142.

Gallaudet University: Founded in 1817 and located in Washington, D.C. It is the only liberal arts college for the deaf in the world.

handicapped: Having some sort of disability, including physical disabilities, mental retardation, sensory impairments, behavioral disorders, learning disabilities or multiple handicaps.

hemiplegia: Paralysis of one side of the body.

inclusion: An educational philosophy that values placing any child with a disability in a regular classroom. This choice is made instead of placing the child in a segregated classroom with other children who have disabilities.

individualized education program (IEP): A written plan that describes what services a local education agency has promised to provide for the child.

individualized family service plan (IFSP): A written document that describes what services the child will receive through an early intervention program.

interdisciplinary team: A team of professionals from different areas of expertise who evaluate the child and develop a comprehensive plan for services which emphasize the child's strengths and needs.

least restrictive environment: The requirement under Public Law 94-142 that children receiving special education must be made a part of a regular school to the fullest intent.

lupus: A chronic inflammatory disease of connective tissue that causes injury to the skin, joints, kidneys, nervous system and mucous membranes.

mainstreaming: The practice of involving children with disabilities in regular school.

microcephaly: A condition in which head circumference is more than two standard deviations below the average size.

Medicaid: A joint state and federal program that offers medical assistance to people who are entitled to receive Supplemental Security Income.

Medicare: A federal program that provides medical care to people who receive Supplemental Security Income.

mental retardation: Having below normal mental function. Children who are mentally retarded learn more slowly than other children. Mental retardation does not indicate a specific level of mental ability. The level of mental function may not be identifiable until later.

motor delay: Having slower than normal development of movement skills.

muscle tone: The amount of tension or resistance to movement in a muscle.

nemaline myopathy: Congenital disease of the skeletal muscles, marked by delayed walking and mild proximal muscle weakness that is not progressive.

occupational therapist: A professional who evaluates and facilitates the development of fine motor skills.

orthotist: Person who creates orthopedic devices (orthoses), most commonly splints or braces, used to support, align or correct deformities or to improve the function of the limbs.

physical therapist: A therapist who works with motor skills.

Glossary

Public Law 94-142: Education for All Handicapped Children Act. The federal law that guarantees all children with disabilities the right to free, appropriate public education.

Public Law 99-457: This law mandates early intervention programs for preschoolers with developmental disabilities.

receptive language: The ability to understand spoken and written communication as well as gestures.

related services: These include services that enable a child to benefit from special education. Related services include occupational, physical and speech therapy, as well as transportation services.

respite care: Skilled adult or child care and supervision that can be provided in the client's home or the home of a care provider.

rheumatoid arthritis: This is a chronic, systemic disease characterized by inflammatory changes in joints and related structures that result in crippling deformity.

rubella: German measles.

seizure: Involuntary movement or changes in consciousness or behavior brought on by abnormal bursts of electrical activity in the brain.

self-help: Relating to skills such as eating, bathing, dressing and cleaning, which enable a person to take care of himself.

spastic diplegia: A type of cerebral palsy with increased muscle tone resulting in stiff movements. It primarily affects the legs.

special education: Specialized instruction based on educational disabilities determined by a team evaluation. It must be matched to the educational needs of the child and adapted to learning style.

special needs: Needs of a person who has a disability.

speech therapist: A specialist who diagnoses and provides treatment for speech, language and listening disorders.

social ability: The ability to function in groups and to interact with others.

Social Security Disability Insurance (SSDI): This is money that has been paid into the Social Security System through payroll deductions. Disabled workers are entitled to these benefits. People who become disabled before the age of twenty-two may collect this under a parent's account if the parent is retired, disabled or deceased.

Supplemental Security Income (SSI): This is available to low-income people who are disabled, blind or aged. This is based on need, not on past earnings.

telecommunications device (TDD): This device allows people who are deaf to talk to non-deaf people over the telephone lines using a small terminal with a screen and an abbreviated keyboard.

thalidomide: A chemical substance used extensively as a sedative and sleeping pill in the early 1960s. Its use was discontinued when it was discovered to cause severe malformations in limbs of developing fetuses exposed to the drug during early intrauterine life. It causes thalidomide syndrome.

vocational training: Training for a job. Learning skills to perform in the work place.

RESOURCE GUIDE

NATIONAL ORGANIZATIONS

Accent on Information
P.O. Box 700
Bloomington, IL 61702
309-378-2961
Will provide information on daily care, products and publications.

Administration on Developmental Disabilities
Department of Health and Human Services
200 Independence Avenue, S.W.
Washington, D.C. 20201
202-690-6590

Alexander Graham Bell Association for the Deaf
3417 Volta Place, N.W.
Washington, D.C. 20007
202-337-5220

American Academy for Cerebral Palsy
1308 Sherwood Avenue
Richmond, VA 23220
804-321-6666

American Association of University Affiliated
Program for Persons with Developmental Disabilities
8630 Fenton Street
Suite 410
Silver Springs, MD 20910
301-588-8252
They will provide you with a list of all national University Affiliated programs which help families with diagnosis and treatment.

American Cleft Palate Foundation
1829 East Franklin Street
Suite 1022
Chapel Hills, NC 27514
800-242-5338
800-24CLEFT

American Council for the Blind
1155 15th Street, N.W.
Suite 720
Washington, D.C. 20005
202-467-5081

American Diabetes Association
National Center
1660 Duke Street
Alexandria, VA 22314
703-549-1500
800-676-4065

American Occupational Therapy Association
P.O. Box 1725, 1383 Piccard Drive
Rockville, MD 20850
301-943-9626
A professional organization which can refer families to local occupational therapists in their area.

Resource Guide

American Physical Therapy Association
1111 N. Fairfax Street
Alexandria, VA 22314
703-684-2782
They can refer families to local physical therapists, as well as provide publications.

American Speech, Language and Hearing Association
10801 Rockville Pike
Rockville, MD 20852
301-897-5700
800-638-8255
They can conduct research regarding communication disorders. They can send publications, make local referrals, and information on software for computers and augmentative communication.

American Orthotic and Prosthetic Association
1650 King Street, Suite 500
Alexandria, VA 22314
703-836-7116

Arthritis Foundation
1330 West Peach Tree Street
Atlanta, GA 30309
800-283-7800

Association for Children and Adults with Learning Disabilities
4156 Library Road
Pittsburgh, PA 15234
412-341-1515
They will refer families to their local chapter.

Association for Children with Down Syndrome, Inc.
2616 Martin Avenue
Bellmore, NY 11710
516-221-4700

Association for Education and Rehabilitation of the Blind and Visually Impaired
4600 Duke Street
Suite 430
P.O. Box 22397
Alexandria, VA 22304
703-823-9690

The Arc: a nonprofit organization on mental retardation
500 East Border Street
Suite 300
Arlington, TX 76010
800-435-5255
817-261-6003

Autism Society of America (ASA)
7910 Woodmont Avenue
Suite 650
Bethesda, MD 20814
800-3-Autism
301-657-0881

Canine Companions For Independence
P.O. Box 446
Santa Rosa, CA 95402
800-572-BARK
707-528-0830

Down Syndrome League
3321 Montevideo Drive
San Ramon, CA 94583
510-556-1700

Epilepsy Foundation of America
4351 Garden City Drive
Landover, MD 20785
301-459-3700
800-EFA-1000

Resource Guide

Federation for Children with Special Needs
312 Stuart Street
Boston, MA 02116
617-482-2915

Heath Resource Center
One Dupont Circle, N.W., Suite 780
Washington, D.C. 20036-1193
800-544-3284
202-939-9320
Higher education and adult training for people with disabilities; clearinghouse on post-secondary education.

IBM National Support Center for Persons With Disabilities
P.O. Box 2150
Alanta, GA 30055
800-IBM-2133
This is an information clearinghouse for adaptive and technical equipment.

Learning Disability Association
4156 Library Road
Pittsburgh, PA 15234
412-341-1515
They provide referrals to local associations, publictions, advocacy and school programs.

March of Dimes Birth Defects Foundation
1275 Mamoroneck Avenue
White Plains, NY 10605
914-428-7100
Publishes many brochures of interest to families with children who have special needs.

Muscular Dystrophy Association
10 East 40th Street
New York, NY 10019
212-689-9040

National Amputation Foundation
1245 150th Street
Flushing, NY 11357
718-767-8400

National Association of the Deaf
814 Thayer Avenue
Silver Springs, MD 20710
301-587-1788
301-587-1791 fax

National Braille Press
88 Saint Stephen Street
Boston, MA 02115
617-437-0456

National Center for Youth with Disabilities
University of Minnesota
P.O. Box 721
Minneapolis, MN 55455
612-625-5000

National Council of Independent Living Centers
310 Laclede Avenue
St. Louis, MO 63108

National Down Sydrome Society
666 Broadway
New York, NY 10012
212-460-9330

National Easter Seal Society
230 West Monroe
Chicago, IL 60606
312-726-6200
They offer public education, screening, advocacy and publications. Each state has its own office.

Resource Guide

National Federation of the Blind
1800 Johnson Street
Baltimore, MD 21230
410-659-9314

National Information Center for Children and Youth with Disabilities
P.O. Box 1492
Washington, D.C. 20013
202-884-8200
800-695-0285

National Information Clearinghouse for Infants with Disabilities
1244 Blossom Street
Columbia, SC 29208

National Information Center on Deafness
Gallaudet University
800 Florida Avenue, N.E.
Washington, D.C. 20542
202-651-5052
202-651-5000
They offer information, publications on deafness, and pre-college programs.

National Institute of Health
Route 355, Mannakee Street
Rockville, MD 20850
301-496-9228

National Lekotek Center
2100 Ridge Avenue
Evanston, IL 60204
There are close to 50 centers nationwide. They offer play, toys and support for families with children with special needs. Call a local United Cerebral Palsy Center in areas to find a Lekotek center in your area.

National Organization for Rare Disorders
P.O. Box 8923
New Fairfield, CT 06812
203-746-6518

National Organization of Disability
910 16th Street, N.W.
Washington, D.C. 20006
202-293-5960

National Rehabilitation Association
633 South Washington Street
Alexandria, VA 22314
703-836-0850

National Spinal Cord Injury Association
8300 Colesville Road, Suite 551
Silver Springs, MD 20910
301-588-6959

United Cerebral Palsy Association
1600 L Street, N.W., Suite 700
Washington, D.C. 20036
800-USA-5-UCP

United States Department of Education
Office of Special Education
Room 3132
330 C Street, S.W.
Washington, D.C. 20202
202-724-4256

United States Department of Health and Human Services
Office of Child Development
200 Independence Avenue, S.W.
Washington, D.C. 20201
202-690-6590

Resource Guide

United States Department of Health and Human Services
Rehabilitation Service Administration
200 Independence Avenue, S.W.
Washington, D.C. 20201
202-690-6590

YOUTH SERVICES

Coalition on Sexuality and Disability
122 East 23rd Street
New York, NY 10010
212-243-3900

Council for Exceptional Children
1920 Association Drive
Reston, VA 22091
703-620-3660
They provide information on the educational needs of children with disabilities.

Global Teen Club International
3120 Oak Road, Suite 309
Walnut Creek, CA 94596
Write for information regarding receiving this newsletter which connects youth with disabilities internationally.

National Center for Youth with Disabilities
University of Minnesota
Box 721
420 Delaware Street S.E.
Minneapolis, MN 55455
612-626-2825
Provides Cydline reviews and Connections newsletters.

Resource Guide

National Information Center for Children and Youth with Disabilities
P.O. Box 1492
Washingon, D.C. 20013
800-999-5599
702-893-6061
Bibliography, A guide to Children's Literature for Disabilities.

Planned Parenthood Federation
1120 Connecticut Ave., N.W.
Washington, D.C. 20036
202-785-3351

Sex Information and Education Council of the United States
130 W. 42nd Street, Suite 2500
New York, NY 10036
212-819-9770

National Mental Health Association
1021 Prince Street
Alexandria, VA 22314
703-684-7722

FAMILY SUPPORT SERVICES

American Self-Help Clearinghouse
Northwest Covenant Medical Center
25 Pocono Road
Denville, NJ 07834
Provides current information and contacts for national self-help groups.

Direct Link For the Disabled
P.O. Box 1036
Solvang, CA 93464

Family Voices
P.O. Box 769
Algodones, NM 87001
505-867-2368
Provides information about national healthcare reform.

Family Resource Center on Disabilities
20 East Jackson Boulevard
Chicago, IL 60604
312-939-3513
Provides information, training manuals, support, publications and newsletter.

Resource Guide

Mothers United for Moral Support
150 Cluster Court
Green Bay, WI 54301
414-336-5333
Families of care-givers of children with any disability, chromosome abnormality or health condition. They provide support to parents by networking and matching parents with similar conditions.

National Fathers Network
c/o Kindering Center
16120 N.E. 8th Street
Bellevue, WA 98008
206-747-4004
Network which develops support programs for fathers and families, mentoring projects, curriculum materials, a quarterly publication.

National Parent Network
1727 King Street, Suite 305
Alexandria, VA 22314
703-684-6763
They provide information about local support groups, share information and resources to promote and support the power of parents to influence and affect policy issues concerning the needs of individuals with disabilities, newsletter.

National Self-Advocacy Organization
Self-Advocates Becoming Empowered in the U.S.
c/o People First of Nebraska
2501 North Street, Suite 411
Lincoln, NE 68510
They provide a list of self-advocacy groups for people with developmental disabilities throughout the United States.

Sibling Information Network
The University of Connecticut
Connecticut's University Affiliated Program on Developmental
    Disabilities
Department of Educational Psychology
24a Glenbrook Road
Box U-64
Storrs, CT 06268

Siblings Support Project
P.O. Box 5371, CL-09
Seattle, WA 98105-0371
206-368-4911

The Pittsburgh Sibling Handbook
Easter Seal Society of Allegheny County
632 Fort Duquesne Boulevard
Pittsburgh, PA 15222
Write to address and they will mail a sibling handbook with helpful information.

ACTIVITIES, RECREATION AND SPORTS

Annual Special Needs Camp Guide
200 Park Avenue South, Suite 816
New York, NY 10003
Write to above address and request guide.

Boy Scouts of America
Scouting for People with Disabilities Program
1325 Walnut Hill Lane
P.O Box 15207
Irving, TX 75015
972-580-2000

Girl Scouts Of America
Scouting for People with Disabilities Program
420 5th Avenue
New York, NY 10022
212-852-8071

Guide to Summer Residential Programs for Individuals with Disabilities
Information Center for Individuals with Disabilities
20 Park Plaza, Suite 330
Boston, MA 02116

North American Riding for the Handicapped Association
P.O. Box 33150
Denver, CO 80233
303-452-1212
Request information about state and local chapters.

Parents Guide to Accredited Camps
American Camping Association
Bradford Woods
500 State Road 67 North
Martinsville, IN 46151

Residential Camping Programs List
National Easter Seal Society
2023 West Ogden Avenue
Chicago, IL 60612

Special Olympics International
1325 G Street, N.W.
Washington, D.C. 20005
202-628-3630
Request state programs and information. Provides sporting opportunities for persons with mental retardation year-round. For adults and children eight years of age. Training for 5-7 year olds.

United States Association for Blind Athletes
33 North Institute Street
Colorado Springs, CO 80903
719-630-0422
Request local information, fact sheets, newsletter.

Very Special Arts
1300 Connecticut Avenue, N.W., Suite 700
Washington, D.C. 20036
800-933-8721
202-737-0645
Provides learning opportunities through the arts for people with disabilities, especially children and youth.

Waterskiing for the People with Physical Disabilities
Mission Bay Aquatic Center
1001 Santa Clara Point
Mission Beach, CA 92109
619-488-1036

Resource Guide

Wheelchair Sports, USA
3595 E. Fountain Boulevard, Suite 1
Colorado Springs, CO 80910
719-574-1150
Request information regarding programs. They provide information about local resources throughout the United States.

Winners on Wheels/Quickie Designs
2842 Business Park Avenue
Fresno, CA 93727
202-292-2171
Ages 7-15 learn to solve problems and take risks in a safe learning environment while building self-esteem. They will send information regarding setting up a local Winners on Wheels chapter.

ADVOCACY, FUTURE PLANNING, DISABILITY AWARENESS

Advocacy, Inc.
7700 Chevy Chase Drive, Suite 300
Austin, TX 78752
512-454-4816

American Bar Association Center
1800 M Street, N.W., Suite 30
Washington, D.C. 20036
202-662-1000

Americans with Disabilities Hotline
800-4664-ADA
Questions and referrals regarding disability rights.

Children's Defense Fund
125 E Street, N.W.
Washington, D.C. 20001
202-628-8787

Disability Rights Education and Defense Fund
2212 6th Street
Berkeley, CA 94710
510-644-2555
Information about civil rights, disability laws and policies; publishes "Disability Rights Now."

Resource Guide

Equal Employment Opportunity Commission
1801 L Street, N.W.
Washington, D.C. 20507
202-275-7377

Estate Planning for Persons with Disabilities
16516 East Alamo Place
Aurora, CO 80015

Federal Student Financial Aid
Office of Student Financial Assistance
P.O. Box 84
Washington, D.C. 20004
There are no special federal financial aid programs to assist individuals with disabilities to attend college, except when a state vocational rehabilitation agency has determined that the best preparation for a job for an individual with a disability is a college education. In these cases, financial assistance may be provided. There are other types of federal financial aid programs which are available to all students in need: grants, loans, work study programs, GI bill, Social Security or GI benefits.

Index of Resource Materials on Fair Housing for People with Disabilities
Community Watch
1101 15th Street, N.W.
Washington, D.C. 20005

Kids on the Block
9385-C Gerwig
Columbia, MD 21046
800-368-KIDS
Thirty-seven programs specific to the disability, disability awareness, social issues, referral to local area of residences; puppets are used to teach people about differences.

Making Your Case
Minnesota Governor's Planning Council on Developmental Disabilities
300 Centennial Office Building
658 Cedar Street
St. Paul, MN 55155
They provide a 32-page booklet on how to influence lawmakers and policy.

National Association of Protection and Advocacy Systems
900 Second Street, N.W., Suite 211
Washington, D.C. 20002

National Organization on Disability
910 16th Street, N.W., Suite 600
Washington, D.C. 20006
202-293-5960
Promotes the acceptance and full participation of the disabled in all aspects of life. Founded in 1982, NOD is the only national disability organization concerned with all disabilities, all age groups and all disability issues.

National Organization on Disability Religion and Disability Program
910 16th Street N.W., Suite 600
Washington, D.C. 20006
202-293-5960
Two pamphlets ("Loving Justice" and "That All May Worship") assist churches and synagogues in providing a warmer welcome to people with disabilities.

National Easter Seal Society Communications Department
230 West Monroe, Suite 1800
Chicago, IL 60606
312-726-6200
Publications and products catalogue, disability awareness community programs, elementary school disability awareness program called "Friends Who Care."

Resource Guide

The Networking Project for People with Disabilities
YWCA of the City of New York
610 Lexington Avenue
New York, NY 10022
212-735-9766

How to set up the Networking Project: A replication packet which includes materials that describe how your community can set up a networking project, including a community advisory board, networks of disabled women and girls, networking conferences and follow-up mentoring activities. "You can Serve Disabled Young Women: Mainstreaming Ideas" and a video-tape called "Positive Images: Portraits of Women with Disabilities."

Social Security Programs
Supplmental Security Income (SSI)
800-772-1213

They will give local information pertaining to services. They provide monthly assistance for children with disabilities. If child qualifies for SSI, he/she qualifies for medicaid. State "intent to file" for benefits when speaking with Social Security Office. If child qualifies for medicaid, the family can also request Early and Periodic Screening, Diagnosis, and Treatment (EPSDT) through the medicaid office. Family must request EPSDT services to find out about eligibility.

CATALOGUES, EQUIPMENT, OTHER READING

Adaptability Products for Rehabilitation and Therapy
P.O. Box 515
Colchester, CT 06415
Home accessories, personal care, adaptive clothing, reachers, wheelchair accessories, mobility, communication and computer access.

AT&T National Special Needs Center
800-233-1222
Offers telephone related services for people with hearing, speech and motion impairments.

Communications/Therapy Skill Builders Materials Catalogue
3830 East Bellevue
P.O. Box 42050
Tucson, AZ 85733
For parents and professionals of children ages birth through five. Offers equipment, feeding oral motor supplies, school readiness equipment and literature.

Disabled Children's Relief Fund
402 Pennsylvania Avenue
Freeport, NY 11520
516-377-1605
Provides equipment, rehabilitation services and prostheses. Request grant information.

Resource Guide

Don Johnson Developmental Equipment, Inc.
Specializing in Communication and Computer Access Catalogue
P.O. Box 639
1000 North Rand Road
Wauconda, IL 60084

Exceptional Parent Library
120 Sylvan Avenue
Englewood Cliff, NJ 07632
201-947-7995
For parents, professionals, caregivers of children and young adults with disabilities. They have library books for families to borrow.

Exceptional Parent Magazine
P.O. Box 3000
Department EP
Denville, NJ 07834
800-562-1973
A magazine published 12 times per year for parents, professionals, caregivers of children and young adults with disabilities.

IBM Corporation National Support Center for Persons with Disabilities
Box C-1030
Atlanta, GA 30005
Compatible computer accessories and software for children with special needs.

Sammons Catalogue
Orthopedic and ADL Products
P.O. Box 386
Western Springs, IL 60558
They offer daily living products.

Special Needs Project Catologue
3463 State Street, Suite 282
Santa Barbara, CA 93105
They offer books about disabilities.

Woodbine House Special Needs Collection
6510 Bells Mill Road
Bethesda, MD 20817
800-847-7323
They publish books about disabilities.

RESIDENTIAL RESOURCES

ANCOR American Network of Community Resources and Options
4200 Evergreen Lane, Suite 315
Annandale, VA 22003
703-642-6614

National Association of Private Schools for Exceptional Children
1522 K Street, N.W.
Washington, D.C. 20009
202-408-3338

ADOPTION RESOURCES

National Adoption Clearinghouse
1930 17th Street, N.W.
Washington, D.C. 20009
202-328-8072

Up With Down Syndrome Foundation
9270 Hammocks Boulevard, Suite 301
Miami, FL 33196
305-386-9115

BIBLIOGRAPHY

1. Marvin A. Fishman, *Pediatric Neurology* (Florida Grune and Stratton, 1986): 57.

2. Leo Buscaglia, *The Disabled and Their Parents, a Counseling Challenge* (New York: Holt and Rinehart and Winston, 1994): 47, 64, 178-199, 386.

3. Siegfried M. Pueschel, M.D., James C. Bernier, MSW, and Leslie E. Weidenmann Ph.D., *The Special Child* (Maryland: Paul H. Brookes, 1988): 15-29.

4. H. Rutherford Turnball, Anne P. Turnball, G.J. Bronicki, Jean Ann Summers and Constance Roeder-Gordon, *Disability and The Family: A Guide to Decisions For Adulthood* (Maryland: Paul H. Brookes, 1989): 107-114.

5. Turnball, Ibid.

6. *The Americans with Disabilities Act Questions and Answers.* (U.S. Department of Justice Civil Rights Division, Sept., 1992)

7. Reed Martin, "Pathways" (Houston, Texas, Oct. 1994): vol. 8, No. 4.

8. Ginny Thornburgh, Anne Rose Davie, "Loving Justice" (Washington, D.C. National Organization on Disability, 1994): 9-11.

9. Charles Meyer, *Surviving Death: A Practical Guide For The Dying and Bereaved* (Connecticut: Twenty-Third Publications, 1988): 80-86.

10. Meyer, Ibid.

11. Meyer, Ibid.

12. Meyer, Ibid.

13. Meyer, Ibid.

14. Dolores Curran, *Stress and Healthy Family* (Minnesota: Winston Press, 1985): 6-28.

15. Curran, Ibid.

16. Robert Veninga, *A Gift Of Hope* (Boston: Little, Brown and Company, 1985): 60-138.

17. Stanley D. Klein and Maxwell J. Shleifer, *It Isn't Fair, Siblings of Children with Disabilities* (Connecticut: Exceptional Parent Press, 1993): 33-45.

18. Debra J. Lobato, *Brothers and Sisters and Special Needs* (Maryland: Paul H. Brookes, 1990): 1-13, 15-42

19. Elaine Geralis, *Children with Cerebral Palsy* (Maryland: Woodbine House, 1993): 44, 144-153.

20. Geralis, Ibid.

21. Irving Dickman and Sol Gordon, *One Miracle at a Time* (New York: Simon and Schuster, 1993): 41-43.

22. "Having a Daughter With A Disability" (Washington: National Information Center for Children and Youth with Handicaps, 1990): Oct., No. 14: 1-13.

Bibliography

23. NICCYH, Ibid.

24. Harilyn Rousso, *Disabled, Female, and Proud* (Connecticut: Exceptional Parent Press, 1993): 1-6.

25. Thomas Lickona, Ph.D., *Raising Good Children From Birth Through The Teenage Years* (New York: Bantam Books, 1983): 181-186.

26. Peggy Finston, M.D., *Parenting Plus—Raising Children With Special Health Needs* (New York: Penguin, 1990): 27-66.

27. Chad Piero, *Talking To Your Child About A Disability*, J.J. Papanikou Center on Special Education and Rehabilitation Kaleidoscope (Connecticut, 1994): vol. 4, No. 2.

28. Finston, Ibid.

29. Gordon, Ibid.: 196-200.

30. Mark L. Batshaw, M.D. and Yvonne M. Perret, M.A., M.S.W., L.C.S.W., *Children with Disabilities, A Medical Primer* (Maryland: Paul H. Brookes, 1992): 571-572.

31. Kay H. Kreigsman, Ph.D., Elinor L. Zaslow, M.A., Jennifer D'Zmura-Rehsteiner, M.A., *Talking Charge-Teenagers Talk About Life And Physical Disabilities* (Maryland: Woodbine House, 1992): 17-20, 25-30.

32. Kriegsman, Ibid.

33. Kriegsman, Ibid.

34. Allison Bell and Lisa Rooney, M.D., *Your Body Yourself—A Guide To Your Changing Body* (Chicago: Contemporary Books, 1993), 131-132.

35. Geralis, Ibid.: 98-304.

36. Geralis, Ibid.: 299.

37. Geralis, Ibid.: 306.

38. Texas Planning Council For Developmental Disabilities.

39. Family to Family News (Houston, Texas), Feb., 1996.

40. Barbara Eberstein, *IEP Strategies,* Exceptional Parent Magazine, 1995: April, 62-63.

41. The National Association of State Directors of Special Education.

42. Dickman, Ibid.: 248-250.

43. Turnball, Ibid.: 84-88.

44. Geralis, Ibid.: 318.

45. Buscaglia, Ibid.: 62-64.

46. Leslie Cogher, Elizabeth Savage, and Michael F. Smith, *Cerebral Palsy The Child and Young Person.* (London: Chapman and Hall Medical, 1992): 42-44.

47. Dickman, Ibid.: 117.